T0265301

OTOLARYNGOLOGY RESEARCH ADVANCES

TONSILLAR DISORDERS: ETIOLOGY, DIAGNOSIS AND TREATMENT

OTOLARYNGOLOGY RESEARCH ADVANCES

Additional books in this series can be found on Nova's website
under the Series tab.

Additional E-books in this series can be found on Nova's website
under the E-books tab.

OTOLARYNGOLOGY RESEARCH ADVANCES

TONSILLAR DISORDERS: ETIOLOGY, DIAGNOSIS AND TREATMENT

ANNE C. HALLBERG
EDITOR

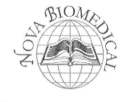

Nova Science Publishers, Inc.

New York

Copyright © 2011 by Nova Science Publishers, Inc.

All rights reserved. No part of this book may be reproduced, stored in a retrieval system or transmitted in any form or by any means: electronic, electrostatic, magnetic, tape, mechanical photocopying, recording or otherwise without the written permission of the Publisher.

For permission to use material from this book please contact us:
Telephone 631-231-7269; Fax 631-231-8175
Web Site: http://www.novapublishers.com

NOTICE TO THE READER

The Publisher has taken reasonable care in the preparation of this book, but makes no expressed or implied warranty of any kind and assumes no responsibility for any errors or omissions. No liability is assumed for incidental or consequential damages in connection with or arising out of information contained in this book. The Publisher shall not be liable for any special, consequential, or exemplary damages resulting, in whole or in part, from the readers' use of, or reliance upon, this material. Any parts of this book based on government reports are so indicated and copyright is claimed for those parts to the extent applicable to compilations of such works.

Independent verification should be sought for any data, advice or recommendations contained in this book. In addition, no responsibility is assumed by the publisher for any injury and/or damage to persons or property arising from any methods, products, instructions, ideas or otherwise contained in this publication.

This publication is designed to provide accurate and authoritative information with regard to the subject matter covered herein. It is sold with the clear understanding that the Publisher is not engaged in rendering legal or any other professional services. If legal or any other expert assistance is required, the services of a competent person should be sought. FROM A DECLARATION OF PARTICIPANTS JOINTLY ADOPTED BY A COMMITTEE OF THE AMERICAN BAR ASSOCIATION AND A COMMITTEE OF PUBLISHERS.

Additional color graphics may be available in the e-book version of this book.

LIBRARY OF CONGRESS CATALOGING-IN-PUBLICATION DATA

Tonsillar disorders : etiology, diagnosis, and treatment / editors, Anne C. Hallberg.
     p. ; cm.
Includes bibliographical references and index.
ISBN 978-1-61209-275-1 (hardcover)
1. Tonsils--Diseases. I. Hallberg, Anne C.
[DNLM: 1. Tonsillitis. WV 430]
RF481.T66 2010
616.3'14--dc22
                                        2010048387

Published by Nova Science Publishers, Inc. † New York

Contents

Preface

This new book discusses the causes of various tonsillar diseases and conditions along with their treatments, including adenoids and related diseases in childhood; markers of lymphoid follicle function in chronic tonsillitis; oral ribosomal immunotherapy in recurrent pharyngotonsillitis; post-tonsillectomy hemorrhage; peritonsillar abscess and tumor necrosis factor producing cells in chronic tonsillitis.

Chapter I - Pediatricians consider adenoiditis, whether it is associated with concomitant obstructive hypertrophy or not, to be one of the most ancient and common problem. Anatomically, adenoids are part of the Waldeyer's ring; and, since they may create mechanical Eustachian Tube (ET) obstruction, they are relevant in the pathogenesis of Otitis Media (OM).

Since 1980, adenoidectomy and sometimes adeno-tonsillectomy are believed to have a role in the management of some patients with OME or recurrent acute OM. The current American Academy of Pediatrics clinical practice guidelines candidate a child for adenoidectomy only in a few cases, unless a distinct indication, namely nasal obstruction, does exist; however, adenoidectomy (with or without concurrent myringotomy) is recommended when children, who have had tympanostomy tube, have OME relapse after tubes extrusion.

ET dysfunction related to adenoids may have also a functional component, potentially allergy-related. Even though the amount of studies over such topic is limited, the interest related to this issue started in 1970, since IgE on mast cells and plasma cells have been demonstrated in adenoid tissue. Nowadays, indeed, allergic adenoiditis indicate a condition in which adenoid tissue exhibit numerous IgE positive mast cells.

In order to diagnose Adenoid hypertrophy or Adenoiditis, nowadays nasal endoscopy is considered to be the gold standard even in young kids, as this technique is also able to detect a possible association between adenoid inflammation/infection and OME, especially during infancy and early childhood.

Chapter II - The lymphoid follicle of palatine tonsil, as a B-cell-rich zone, is the site of proliferation, differentiation and selection of the antigen-stimulated B cells. All of these processes are taking place in specific microenvironment that is product of lymphoid follicle cells.

Methods: The microenvironment of lymphoid follicles was analyzed on tonsillar tissue specimens from patients with recurrent tonsillitis (RT) and hypertrophic tonsillitis (HT). Structural organization of lymphoid follicles was observed by scanning electron microscopy. Proliferation and differentiation of stimulated follicular B cells, as well as apoptotic and inflammatory factors in lymphoid follicles were analyzed by LSAB/HRP method on paraffin slices using monoclonal antibody for Ki-67, Bcl-2, Bax and TNF-α, respectively. The follicular immunoglobulin (Ig) - producing cells were detected by using PAP method. Moreover, we have investigated the enzyme activity of 5′-nukleotidase (5′-NT), Mg^{2+}ATPase and dipeptidyl peptidase IV (DPP IV) using enzymohistochemical and immunohistochemical methods. AgNOR method was performed to determine the cell cycle of the follicular lymphocytes. In addition to this, quantitative Image analysis of lymphoid follicles and follicular cells was also done.

Results: Both types of tonsillitis show similar distribution of Ki-67-, Bcl-2-, Bax- and TNF-α- expressing cells and Ig-producing cells as well, although number of investigated cells was different. The greater number of cells in follicular germinal centers was in G_1 phase, whereas the most of lymphocytes in mantle zone were in $S+G_2$ phase of cell cycle, with significant differences between HT and RT. Activity of 5′-NT, Mg^{2+}ATPase and DPP IV is localized in different morphological compartments of the palatine tonsil, however, each of these enzymes doesn't show the difference in localization between RT and HT.

Conclusion: The numerous factors contribute to specific environment for proliferation and differentiation of stimulated B cells in lymphoid follicles of palatine tonsil. The quantitative differences of investigated markers, used for demonstration of dynamic processes associated with follicular B cells, suggest the different immune response in tonsils with RT compared to that with HT.

Chapter III - Pharyngotonsillitis is a common illness in adults and children, often encountered by family and emergency medicine physicians. An infection in the pharynx, which is served by the lymphoid tissues of Waldeyer's ring, can spread to other parts of the ring, such as the tonsils, nasopharynx, uvula, soft palate, adenoids, and cervical lymph glands, causing pharyngitis, tonsillitis, pharyngotonsillitis, and/or rhinosinusitis. These illnesses can be acute, subacute, chronic, or recurrent.

The reasons for recurrent pharyngotonsillitis are not deeply understood yet. In the last decades several authors have tried to explain how modifications affecting the balance of a host's immunological functions on the one hand and infection agents on the other can lead to recurrent inflammatory events: although much has been written on how to manage recurrent pharyngo-tonsillitis, it remains a controversial topic.

The etiologic agents may be of viral or bacterial origin. Although viruses are the most common agents that cause throat infections in children, about 30% of infections are of bacterial origin. A proper treatment should provide patients with adequate coverage of aerobic as well as anaerobic pathogens so as to minimize recurrences, enhance eradication, maximize compliance and avoid resistance. Because of antibiotic resistance increase, attention has been focused on alternative treatment.

The aim of this chapter is to evaluate the efficiency of an oral ribosomal immunotherapy in the management of patients with recurrent pharyngo-tonsillitis.

Chapter IV - The tonsils, located at the back of the throat, are part of Waldeyer's ring located in the pharynx and the back of the oral cavity. They are considered part of the immune system, which is the primary line of defense against infection by bacteria and viruses. Tonsillar diseases and conditions include infection, cancer, hypertrophied tonsils and "kissing tonsils", and both acute and chronic tonsillar infections are very common in children. This review discusses the causes of various tonsillar diseases and conditions along with their treatments and will also include primary tonsillar infections leading to other morbidities. For example, some tonsillar infections are associated with rheumatic joint and heart conditions. Furthermore, because of the importance of tonsillar function in the overall immune system, the indications for and effects of tonsillectomy will be reviewed.

Chapter V - The most serious complication of tonsillectomy is bleeding. Primary post-tonsillectomy hemorrhage (PTH) occurs during the first 24 hours following the procedure, usually as a consequence of inadequate ligation of the feeding arteries. Secondary PTH occurs most frequently between the 5-8 postoperative days. Incidence of such episodes counts in several percent being an important clinical problem due to the number of tonsillectomies being very

frequently performed ENT procedures. PTH occurs significantly more
frequently in adults (age equal to or above 15 years) than in children. In
children, the risk is higher in boys and in individuals with frequent infections
of the tonsils. In adult patients, peritonsillar abscess as indication for surgery
increases the risk of PTH. Bleeding occurs more frequently after "hot" than
"cold" technique and the use of coblation significantly increases the
occurrence of PTH. Cryptic tonsillitis and actinomyces infection diagnosed on
histopathological examination of tonsillar tissue were found to correlate with
PTH, whereas patient's gender and season of surgery were not. Performing
tonsillectomy in warmer weather when water vapor pressure is higher may
reduce secondary hemorrhage rate. Incidence of secondary PTH does not
depend on post-operative infection. Post-tonsillectomy hemorrhage rate
significantly correlates with personal history of proneness to bruise formation
and proneness to prolonged bleeding after minor injuries. In rare cases, the
intensity of PTH may become life-threatening and requires major surgical
means and intensive care.

Chapter VI - Objective: is to determine and quantify the production of
TNF-α in chronic tonsillitis.

Material and methods: The study comprised of 23 patients with chronic
tonsillitis, divided in two groups: 10 patients with tonsillar hypertrophy (TH)
with average age 9.0 ± 2.7 years, and 13 patients with recurrent tonsillitis (RT)
aged 23.1 ± 5.2 years.

Highly sensitive labeled streptavidin-biotin horse reddish peroxidase
immunohistochemical method (LSAB+/HRP) was used for detection of TNF-
α producing cells. Quantification of TNF-α was made for crypt epithelium,
germinative centers, roundness of follicles, interfollicular areas and
subepithelial area. Quantification of lymph follicles and germinative centers
included: areal (mm2), median optical density (au), circumference (mm),
Ferret diameter (mm), and integrated optical density (IOD).

Results: Distribution of TNF-α producing cells is similar for TH and RT.
They are mainly found in subepithelial areas, interfollicular regions, and
germinative centers of lymph follicles, and rarely in crypt epithelium.
Numerical density of TNF-α producing cells is significantly higher in RT,
compared to TH.

Conclusion: Quantification of TNF-α producing cells confirm domination
of cellular Th1 immune response both in TH and RT.

Short Communication - Peritonsillar abscess (quinsy) is a complication of
acute bacterial tonsillitis. Its treatment remains controversial. Needle drainage
of the abscess may provide an alternative to incision or tonsillectomy. An

important element of controversy is the choice of antibiotics after surgical drainage of the abscess. Results of many studies support the resistance of grown bacteria to many antibiotics and the potential importance of anaerobic bacteria in development of peritonsillar abscesses. Although bacteria grown from the pus vary among the continents, clinical implications resulting from the microbiological studies are similar. Patients with peritonsillar abscesses should be treated with antibiotics effective against both aerobic and anaerobic bacteria.

In the routine management of peritonsillar abscess, bacteriologic studies are unnecessary on initial presentation. It is, however, necessary to consider infection with anaerobes. Therefore, penicillin and metronidazole are recommended as the antibiotic regimen of choice in the treatment of peritonsillar abscesses. If this treatment is ineffective, broad-spectrum antibiotics (clinadmycin) should be administered.

In: Tonsillar Disorders
Editor: Anne C. Hallberg

ISBN: 978-1-61209-275-1
©2011 Nova Science Publishers, Inc.

Chapter I

Adenoids and Related Diseases in Childhood

D. Caimmi, A. Marseglia, E. Labò, E. Borali, G. Ciprandi, A. M. Castellazzi, F. Pagella and G. L. Marseglia[*]

Foundation IRCCS Policlinico San Matteo - University of Pavia,
Pavia, Italy

Abstract

Pediatricians consider adenoiditis, whether it is associated with concomitant obstructive hypertrophy or not, to be one of the most ancient and common problem. Anatomically, adenoids are part of the Waldeyer's ring; and, since they may create mechanical Eustachian Tube (ET) obstruction, they are relevant in the pathogenesis of Otitis Media (OM).

Since 1980, adenoidectomy and sometimes adeno-tonsillectomy are believed to have a role in the management of some patients with OME or recurrent acute OM. The current American Academy of Pediatrics clinical practice guidelines candidate a child for adenoidectomy only in a

[*] Prof. Gian Luigi MARSEGLIA, MD (Corresponding Author), Department of Pediatric Sciences, Foundation IRCCS Policlinico San Matteo - University of Pavia, P.le Golgi, 2 - 27100 Pavia, Italy, e-mail: gl.marseglia@smatteo.pv.it, tel: +39 0382 502583 fax: +39 0382 527976

few cases, unless a distinct indication, namely nasal obstruction, does exist; however, adenoidectomy (with or without concurrent myringotomy) is recommended when children, who have had tympanostomy tube, have OME relapse after tubes extrusion.

ET dysfunction related to adenoids may have also a functional component, potentially allergy-related. Even though the amount of studies over such topic is limited, the interest related to this issue started in 1970, since IgE on mast cells and plasma cells have been demonstrated in adenoid tissue. Nowadays, indeed, allergic adenoiditis indicate a condition in which adenoid tissue exhibit numerous IgE positive mast cells.

In order to diagnose Adenoid hypertrophy or Adenoiditis, nowadays nasal endoscopy is considered to be the gold standard even in young kids, as this technique is also able to detect a possible association between adenoid inflammation/infection and OME, especially during infancy and early childhood.

Anatomy of the Adenoids

Nasal-associated lymphoid tissues are major inductive organs in the mucosal immune system of the upper respiratory tract [1]. These tissues are localized in a strategic position, in order to mediate local and regional immune functions, as they are exposed both to outside air antigens and to alimentary antigens. Adenoids have characteristics similar to lymphoid glands, and, together with tonsils, are part of the mucosa-associated lymphoid tissues, having a major role in the induction of immunity. Indeed, they actually play a main role as effector organs in both mucosal-type and systemic-type adaptive immunity [2].

The Waldeyer's ring is formed by lymphoid tissue and it consists superiorly of the pharyngeal tonsils, also known as the adenoids; laterally of the two palatine tonsils, strategically located at the entrance of the oropharynx; and inferiorly of the lingual tonsils located at the base of the tongue [3]. Such immunologically complex structure is prominent mainly during childhood, when it occupies a major part of the oro-nasopharyngeal space, which is not yet fully developed during the first years of life [3]. The lymphoid tissue undergoes hypertrophy and hyperplasia, and it reaches its greatest mass when kids are aged between 2 and 5 years; during puberty, on the other hand, we may assist to its gradual involution [3].

Each adenoid consists of 50–60% B lymphocytes, 40% T lymphocytes, and approximately 3% plasma cells [4]. Adenoids are responsible for *in vivo* immune reactions through non-specific anti-bacterial factors such as mucosal villous transport, mucin, lysozyme, and lactoferrin, and through antibody synthesis [5]. The adenoids provide local secretory IgA, being part of the mucosa-associated lymphoid tissues, and thus presenting patches of respiratory-type secretory epithelium on their surface and crypts [6]. It is known that adenoidal tissue, because of peculiar location is constantly exposed to allergens [7]. IgA plays, therefore, a major role in mucosal immunity in the adenoids, binding to bacteria and suppressing bacterial colonization in the epithelium, thus blocking microbial toxins and other antigens. Mucus is transported from the nasal cavity and paranasal sinuses directly towards the adenoid. Secondary to ciliary movement, the proportion of allergen reaching the mucous membrane is moved to the nasopharyngeal cavity and then to the pharynx where it is then swallowed [7].

IgA comprises approximately 15–20% of serum antibody [8], and secretory IgA (sIgA) on the mucosal surface, in particular, plays an important role in immunity [9]. IgA precursor cells are formed in the adenoids and then distributed to other reactive tissues and organs [6,10]. A reduction in serum IgA may be outlined in those patients who seem to be easily susceptible to recurrent infections [11]. In normal conditions, the active interaction, between innate and adaptive immunity, and with nonspecific mechanical factors, may be able to contribute to the prevention of microorganism invasion. This interaction is partly caused by Toll-like receptors (TLRs), that may, nonetheless, be reduced in those children with recurrent respiratory infections or exposed to passive smoke, suggesting therefore a crucial immunological function played by TLRs in upper airway diseases [12]. Moreover, in children exposed to passive smoke, a reduction of Th1 adenoidal lymphocytes (IFNγ-CD8+) can be detected and it becomes even more evident in those patients presenting with recurrent respiratory infections [13].

Such reduction may bring to a decreased immunity to viruses, bacteria, and other antigens, and to an increased chance to develop Otitis Media with Effusion (OME) or Chronic Rhinosinusitis (CRS) [1].

Moreover, it has to be underlined that deeply, the lymphoid tissue is characterized by the presence of follicular germinal centers and interfollicular areas, which are predominantly populated by T-lymphocytes. The localization and function of effector T-cells is crucial to generate an effective immune response. In particular, CD8+ T lymphocytes can mobilize two main mechanisms: cytolysis and production of cytokines, chemokines and micro-bicidal molecules. If the production of IFN-gamma is reduced, patients show an increased susceptibility to infectious viral diseases, which often precede upper respiratory tract infections, with a possible consequential increase in replication of pathogenic bacteria in the adenoidal tissue [14].

Being adenoids as reservoirs of viruses and bacteria, it has to be underlined that infections may contribute both to Eustachian tube dysfunction and to tissue hypertrophy.

The Eustachian tube (ET) provides an anatomic communication between middle ear cavity and nasopharynx, and it is usually collapsed, protecting middle ear from nasal contents [15]. In pathological conditions, negative pressure resulting from middle ear hypoventilation produces alterations of gas exchanges with mucosal epithelium and, as a consequence, transudation of fluid, with a major risk of developing Otitis Media [15].

One of the main problems concerning adenoidal tissue in childhood is related to adenoidal hypertrophy (AH). Lymphoid hyperplasia appears to be due to an increase in lymphoid elements., and it is directly proportional to the mean bacterial load [16]. Of the different pathogens, mainly Haemophilus influenzae and Staphylococcus aureus have been associated with lymphoid hyperplasia [17,18]. These two bacteria might therefore play an etiologic role in the development of lymphoid hyperplasia [3]. The distribution of dendritic cells, which are antigen presenting cells, has been shown to be altered during disease [19,20]. There is a correlation between the bacterial load and the frequency of dendritic cells in these areas [20], indicating that the body adapts to better defend against invading micro-organisms.

AH, as tonsillar hypertrophy too, may affect kids in different ways resulting in: Eustachian tube dysfunction/otitis media; rhinosinusitis; obstructive sleep apnea; facial growth abnormalities; swallowing problems; reduced ability to smell and taste; speech problems; and affect overall quality of life [3].

Adenoiditis and Otitis Media

Morphological studies on adenoids suggest a connection between the mucociliary transport system, the secretory structures, and the infectious and immunological events and the pathogenesis of Otitis Media (OM) [21]. OM is a disease characterized by the inflammation of the middle ear: it can occur at any age, but the population affected the most is composed by infants and children [15]. From a clinical point of view, OM is usually classified into acute OM (AOM), recurrent acute OM, OM with effusion (OME) and chronic suppurative OM. AOM is defined as a history of acute onset of signs and symptoms of middle ear inflammation, usually accompanied by the presence of middle ear effusion, which can take some weeks to be reabsorbed [22]. AOM is recurrent when these episodes are not isolated, namely with an incidence of 3 in six months or 4 in one year, approximately [22]. OME is a form lacking acute clinical manifestations of inflammation, but it is characterized by the persistent presence of fluid in middle ear cavity, which can affect seriously child hearing function [22]. Chronic Otitis media with effusion (COME) is the most common chronic ear disorder in children. COME is defined as the persistence of middle ear fluid beyond 12 weeks and has multiple causes, including environmental and host factors. [23]

Medical treatment (including eradication of upper respiratory tract infections, control of allergy, and environmental precautions) is the first choice of management, followed by ventilation tube insertion and/or adenoidectomy [23].

The etiology of OM in children is complex, resulting from a combination of several endogenous and exogenous factors, including biofilm formation, infections, and Eustachian Tube dysfunction.

In most cases of OME, middle ear fluid does not show bacterial growth and, furthermore, antibiotic therapy usually doesn't result in any significant benefit for its resolution [24]. However, the presence of bacteria into organized and complex aggregates, named as biofilms, provides more resistance to bacteria, against host immunological defenses and antibiotics, and it may promote recurrence or persistence of OM [25]. The role of biofilms has been studied and investigated mainly in recent years, as they have been considered as a great component in the explanation of chronic infections and resistance to antibiotic chemotherapy. Indeed, biofilms play a major role in the formation of many chronic or recurrent diseases. This is true in ENT disorder too: in facts, otitis media, sinusitis, cholesteatoma, tonsillitis, adenoiditis, and device infections may be all related to the existence of a biofilm layer. Such thin layer is composed of bacteria encased in a hydrated matrix of polysaccharide and protein, which is able to adhere to all surface tissues [23]. When the layer begins to form, the bacterial attachment is reversible, until bacteria elaborate a glycocalyx, making the adhesion irreversible; afterwards, growth continues by the division of sessile bacteria and the recruitment of other bacteria, forming glycocalyx-enclosed micro-colonies [23]. Biofilm formation is detectable also on adenoid surfaces, particularly in children with recurrent infections [23].

AOM is essentially considered an infectious disease, but ET impairment can play anyway an important role as well; ET dysfunction in this setting seems to arise directly from ongoing infectious process itself. Indeed, AOM is often preceded by a (viral) upper airway infection, resulting in mucosal congestion of nasopharynx and ET and, as a consequence, in mechanical obstruction; the development of middle ear negative pressure results in "aspiration" of pathogens from the nasopharynx into the middle ear cavity and impairment of local mucociliary clearance, which leads to microbial proliferation in middle ear secretions [26]. As for OME, even though a microbial involvement has been recently demonstrated in some studies, OME lacks typical signs and symptoms of acute infectious inflammation, although it can follow one or more episodes of AOM [27]. In COME, on the other hand, the infectious process seems to be maintained by tympanic membrane perforation, which can further promote the access of bacteria from nasopharynx, as middle ear air cushion get lost, in addition to the possibility of contamination from the external ear canal [26].

Obstruction (opening failure) and sometimes abnormal patency of ET have been both suggested to predispose to OM. Obstruction can be mechanical or functional: the former can derive from inflammatory secretions and mucosal edema, extrinsically in posterior nasopharynx or intrinsically in ET, or from enlarged adenoids or nasopharyngeal tumors, for instance [15]. The latter occurs for persistent collapse of ET, due to alterations of wall compliance or inefficient active/muscular opening; this condition appear to be common among infants and younger children: a lesser amount and stiffness of the cartilage support in addition to a lesser efficiency of the muscle is believed to be responsible [15]. Functional and mechanical obstruction can be measured through so-called active and passive function tests, respectively [24]. Functional ET dysfunction is considered essentially an endogenous/ constitutional factor, whereas mechanical ET obstruction derives primarily from viral/bacterial infections of upper respiratory airways, adenoiditis, and nasal inflammation, including also allergic rhinitis (AR) [24]. In facts, inflammation constitutes a constant feature of OME, as well as AOM. However, if in the latter inflammatory changes are clearly elicited by infectious agents, in OME this link is not always evident at all, leading to speculate that its pathogenesis may recognize different mechanisms, instead of or in addition to the presence of bacteria and viruses in middle ear cavity [28].

Evidences that adenoids could be involved in immunological processes occurring mainly in allergic patients and affecting somehow upper respiratory disease (including OME) derives from some studies reporting an alteration of

T cells subsets and especially an increased presence of IgE+ and Fcε-RI+ cells in these patients [29]. Also, there is an increase in the number of lymphocytes, mast cells, plasma cells, macrophages, dendritic cells, and M cells in the adenoids of patients with OME when compared with normal children [21].

It is known that persistent infection lead to epithelial destruction; such eventuality may in turn allow penetration of antigens through the damaged epithelium. Antigens are therefore able to reach lymphocytes, secondarily to the formation of clefts down to the lymphoid tissue, which multiply the immunologic reactions [21]. The infection of the adenoid tissue, or a condition of adenoiditis (infection and/or inflammation) may thus increase the amount of local immune cells, reflecting an increased antigenic load.

In those areas that show degeneration or reparation with collagenous and reticular fibers, dendritic cells are in contact with lymphocytes through their cytoplasmic elongations, which suggests that around these cells, charged to present antigenic stimuli to lymphocytes, there are several antigens and antibodies, able to activate the complement system. When activated, the complement causes vasodilatation, increase in vascular permeability, and fluid exudation, all conditions that can precipitate OME [21].

When a child presents with recurrent episodes of otitis media or with symptoms indicating a possible adenoiditis, a complete medical evaluation should be performed. Clinicians should carefully collect a detailed history of the child, investigate the allergic status of the patient, and advise to perform a nasal endoscopy, in order both to reach a more precise diagnosis and to obtain microbiologic findings. In facts, the abundance of purulent foci despite clinically undetectable infections underlines the need to perform such an examination in this group of patients [30].

Adenoiditis and Allergy

The role of allergy in adenoidal diseases is not clear. Even though there are several different conditions that can lead to AH, it is commonly assumed that chronic, severe and recurrent inflammatory processes concerning the adenoids may be of particular significance. Allergic diseases are, as it seems now obvious, only one manifestation of such inflammation [7]. Recent Literature suggests that in a certain group of children the factor responsible for the occurrence of AH is a coexisting allergic disorder, mostly allergic rhinitis (AR) [31].

Allergic adenoiditis is defined as the presence of numerous brightly fluorescent IgE mast cells demonstrated in formalin-fixed adenoid tissue by the trypsin-immunofluorescent method [32]. In the 1980s, it was shown that, in patients presenting with AR, IgE synthesis was detectable around the Waldeyer's ring and other local lymphnodes; in facts, in the nasal mucosa itself, sensitized mast cells occur already covered by antibodies [33]. Recent studies have pointed out a high affinity with IgE (Fcε-RI) as well as mRNA for IL-4, resulting in an increased receptor expression, demonstrating that in the adenoid tissue there is immunoglobulin class switching to IgE [7].

It is well established that the early years of life are crucial for the development of allergic diseases. Nevertheless, it is not clear which are the factors capable of controlling both the possible manifestation and the seriousness of the clinical manifestations [34]. One of these factors is the allergen sensitization route and the nose plays an important role in the atopic march for airways diseases. A first indication of a potential role for the adenoid during allergic sensitization in the airways are differences cellular and cytokine profiles between allergic and non-allergic children.

In facts, atopic children adenoids may present a more prominent eosinophilic inflammatory pattern than those of non-atopic children [35]. Eosinophils are considered to be one of the major effector cells involved in the allergic inflammation [36]. These cells are usually seen in the mucosa lining the shock organs of allergy (e.g. nasal mucosa and bronchi), and are quickly recruited and activated after a contact with the allergen [37-39]. On the other hand, IgA, particularly secretory IgA, is able to mediate eosinophil degranulation *in vitro* [40] and allergic patients show an increased expression of IgA receptors on their eosinophils [41], proving even more that diseased adenoids have a different cell population than healthy adenoids [42]. Moreover, the inflammation of nasal mucosa, which, as said, is part of the allergic route, may induce specific alterations only in a subgroup of patients, that will later develop OME [43]. An increasing attention have been focused also to a potential role played by adenoids in inducing ET in allergic patients and different studies have concluded that, in patients with ET dysfunction and OME, adenoid tissue contains a significantly increased number of mast cells [43].

The number of atopy-related diseases has been increasing for a fairly long time and Paediatricians are well aware that AR is one of the main manifestations of allergy, especially in younger age groups [44]. It has been assumed that allergic rhinitis may be an important factor responsible for AH [45]. Nevertheless, since in the same age group in which AH show the highest incidence allergic rhinitis occurs relatively rarely, this factor has now bee considered as relevant only for some children. In general, therefore, it cannot be said that AR is the key cause of AH in the general population. It has to be pointed out, though, that the clinical symptoms of allergic rhinitis and AH are similar, and, consequently, it is likely that very often only one disease entity is recognised [31].

Children suffering from specific allergies should experience an enlargement of their adenoidal size during times of exposure to those antigens to which they are sensitized. These size changes could be measured, as well as spirometric values could be too. Such measurements can be easily detected if the patient is sensitized to seasonal allergens, whose exposure period is to a large extent predictable. In the case of perennial allergens that circulate in the air all year long at a similar level of concentration (e.g. dust mites) or occur irregularly inducing chronic allergic rhinitis, such changes could be difficult to be underlined [31].

Nevertheless, dust mites are one of the most frequent perennial sensitizing allergens in Western Countries, having therefore clinical significance. In children with allergic rhinitis related to hypersensitivity to dust mites, adenoid hypertrophy occurs significantly more frequently than in children with other allergic diseases (asthma/atopic dermatitis) or with no allergies [7]. Moreover, in children with AH, a coexisting hypersensitivity to plant pollen allergens and allergens has been proven to be more frequent than in children without AH, showing that, in those areas where such allergens dominate, AR caused by these allergens is the main factor leading to allergic adenoiditis [7].

The exposure to a sensitising factor may therefore be one of the causes responsible for adenoid hypertrophy in children with allergic rhinitis, and an appropriate treatment for AR may reduce the incidence of adenoid hypertrophy in hypersensitive children [31].

The Role of Surgery

Approximately one million adenoidectomy procedures were performed in the United States in the 1970s, but, in these last 20 years, the number of such operations has dramatically decreased, mainly because of the several discussions over the pros and cons for this procedure [21]. Nevertheless, adenoidectomy remains one of the most commonly performed pediatric procedures in the world [46].

In Paediatrics, the most common indications for such procedure include chronic otitis media (often combined with bilateral myringotomy and tubes), medically refractory chronic rhinosinusitis, and airway obstruction (often combined with tonsillectomy) [47].

In patients with healthy ears and adenoid hypertrophy, history of apnea is the main indication for adenoidectomy, together with a high frequency of upper respiratory tract infections [23]. Adenoids removed for airway obstruction and/or recurrent infections have been studied to identify a possible mechanism to explain chronic evolution, and they have shown the presence of bacterial biofilms on their surfaces, mainly in children with concomitant otorrhoea [48].

Adenoid pads can create ET obstruction, when they are enlarged and/or inflamed, because their proximity. Since 1980, adenoidectomy and sometimes adenotonsillectomy are believed to have a role in the management of some patients with OME or recurrent AOM [49]. In those children presenting with medical resistant COME, the treatment include ventilation tube insertion and/or adenoidectomy [50]. The critical question is whether adenoidectomy is effective through removal of mechanical obstruction of eustachian tube or removal of reservoir of chronic infection. In facts, adenoids in COME may act as a reservoir of chronic infection rather than causing mechanical eustachian obstruction [23]. Current AAP clinical practice guidelines candidate a child for adenoidectomy only in a few cases, unless a distinct indication, namely nasal obstruction, does exist; however, adenoidectomy (with or without concurrent myringotomy) is recommended when children who have had tympanostomy tube have OME relapse after tubes extrusion [22]. Effectiveness of this surgery is recognized in children who are at least 3-4 years and older; on the contrary, in younger patients, adenoidectomy (during the insertion of tubes) doesn't seem to be beneficial [51].

Paediatric rhinosinusitis is an important health issue in the pediatric population and outpatient visits for upper respiratory infection are second only to well baby visits amongst primary care providers [52]. Many patients fail conservative medical management, while symptoms improvement can be detected after adenoidectomy for patients suffering from chronic rhinos-inusitis: in facts, these patients report a reduction of rhinorrhea, cough, post-nasal drip, halitosis, as well as of antibiotic prescriptions [47]. Even though there is a consensus favoring surgical intervention in this group of children, there is still disagreement about which type of surgical intervention is appropriate, since both adenoidectomy and endoscopic sinus surgery have both been recommended as surgical options [53]. Some authors suggest that sinus washes through a middle meatal antrostomy should be considered at the time of adenoidectomy, even though the ideal population who would actually benefit from this procedure has not been standardized [54].

It has to be pointed out, though, that certain children undergoing adenotonsillectomy are at markedly increased risk for post-operative airway complications: in facts, infants and toddlers, the morbidly obese, children with cranio-facial abnormalities, hypotonia or failure to thrive, children with severe obstructive sleep apnea by polysomnography are clearly at increased risk for airway obstruction in the immediate perioperative period [55]. Some authors require for such surgeries to be performed at tertiary paediatric hospitals, while some others have suggested a post-operative routine observation in a intensive care unit (ICU) for high-risk patients [56,57].

Moreover, even in normal children, unexpected post-surgery respiratory complications may occur, including post-obstructive pulmonary oedema, pneumonia, and protracted upper airway obstruction from tongue or uvular [58]. Nevertheless, in general, adenoidectomy should be considered as first line surgical therapy for chronic otitis media, medically refractory chronic rhinosinusitis, and airway obstruction, since it is an overall simple, low risk procedure that can easily be performed on an outpatient basis with minimal required post-operative follow-up visits [47].

The Role of Nasal Endoscopy

In a patient presenting with general symptoms of adenoiditis, diagnosis can be challenging. Even though for the diagnosis of adenoid hypertrophy, there are several different recommendations, including lateral neck X-rays, videofluoroscopy, palpation, and nasal endoscopy, the role of each one remains a controversial issue [59].

In general, physicians, despite the wide use of different diagnostic tools in the assessment of adenoid hypertrophy, reach a diagnosis on a clinical basis, since most of the patients complain for snoring, chronic mouth breathing, sleep apnea, and otitis media [59].

Many researchers have tried to identify the most simple, objective, reliable, and minimally invasive mean to evaluate both adenoidal size and adenoid-nasopharynx relation [60]. Since in these past recent years the clinical use of nasal flexible fiberoptic endoscopy has become common, it is currently recommended as the best way to measure adenoidal hypertrophy, and to identify a clinical picture of adenoiditis [61]. In facts, nasal flexible fiberoptic endoscopy (using 2.7-mm rigid endoscopy) can be a tolerable diagnostic tool in children if the procedure is clearly defined for them [59]. The high values of sensitivity and specificity, the agreement of results and the small rate of refusals suggest that nasal endoscopy, besides being helpful in difficult cases, is a highly accurate diagnostic tool, it is safe, objective, and dynamic, and easy to perform in cooperative children [62].

Preoperative evaluations of children with nasal obstruction should be conducted to ensure safe surgical treatments, but nasal endoscopy can be used as a surgical technique as well. Since adenoidectomy is often performed in a hurry, it can be, in many cases, a "Blind Operation". As a result, many children suffer from recurrent adenoiditis or recurrent AH. One of the explanations of such recurrence is ''missing'' adenoid tissue, especially if there are choanal adenoids, at this site; the adenoid tissue is difficult to access by the regular curette, and is difficult to visualize by the mirror [63]. If adenoidectomy is performed endoscopically, there are very few chances that such recurrency may happen, while there is no difference in time and costs for this procedure if compared with other methods used [63].

As a diagnostic tool, further insight have been shed by performing nasal endoscopy in children affected by upper airways respiratory disease: indeed, this procedure allows investigators to visualize adenoids and, in general, rhinopharynx structures directly and in a minimally invasive manner [64]. Identifying the etiology of nasal obstruction in children is an almost daily practice at a pediatric care clinic, but only an accurate diagnosis may be associated to an adequate therapy. Studies have demonstrated that symptoms of nasal obstruction are strongly correlated with adenoid size [62]. Therefore, it is crucial to visualize in the best possible way the adenoidal area, the Waldeyer's ring and the nose.

Inflammation of adenoids seems to be a problem mainly belonging to younger children, maybe because they are more prone to recurrent respiratory infections. Considering the results obtained by nasal endoscopy, it has been possible to prove that OME frequency seems to vary according to the detected pattern, especially in younger age classes, suggesting a role of adenoid disease in the development of OME [65]. Moreover, nasal endoscopy has proven to be very much effective to diagnose acute rhinosinusitis and adenoiditis, and to differentiate between these two diseases: in facts, the clinical features of adenoiditis are very similar to those of acute rhinosinusitis, especially in younger children; actually, the symptoms of these conditions may in some cases overlap and there is no pathognomonic sign [64]. In these cases nasal endoscopy is able to better visualize the adenoid area. In facts, nasal flexible fiberoptic endoscopy makes it possible o visualize adenoids and, in general, rhinopharynx structures directly and in a minimally invasive manner and to distinguish between pictures of isolated rhinosinusitis, isolated adenoiditis or concomitant patterns [66].

Conclusions

Even when presenting with adenoid hypertrophy, not all children develop symptoms. The question remains whether the enlargement of the lymphoid tissue causes obstruction in a normal space, or if in some children the physiological reduction in the dimension of the anatomical space causes the typical feature. In general though, it seems that adenoid hyperplasia, rather than a decreased nasopharyngeal space, is the main cause of nasopharyngeal obstruction in young children. A decreased pharyngeal diameter and a shorter soft palate combined with an increased volume of the tonsils may be the cause of airway obstruction. Infections and allergic inflammation are most likely the possible etiologic factors in lymphoid hyperplasia.

Adenoid tissues of patients with OME seem to be infectious foci, aggravating immune reactions, which might attack the middle ear through an ascending route. The idea that adenoids can worsen middle ear disease has been proposed for decades, especially when it is not a simple hypertrophy, but there is clear inflammation/infection (adenoiditis). Indeed, adenoids can serve as reservoir of bacterial pathogen infecting middle ear, not only for chronic otitis, but also with respect to OME. H. influenzae and S. aureus are the germs found the most in kids presenting with adenoiditis. Their important role may be also explained by the fact that these bacteria are more prone to resist to medical treatment by forming biofilms on the adenoids surface, so that the purulent process often persists during asymptomatic periods of adeno-tonsillitis, perpetuating the local inflammation.

Moreover, adenoiditis has been considered as potential site of allergic inflammation, which may provide a further link between allergy, especially AR, and OME. In facts, in adenoidal tissue, it is possible to detect an increased number of IgE on mast cells and plasma cells, so that the term "allergic adenoiditis" can now be used to indicate a condition in which adenoid tissue exhibit numerous IgE positive mast cells. The presence of AR increases the likelihood of AH occurrence in children, but at the same time it does not mean that it is its main cause. Similar effects can be induced by any other inflammatory process in the vicinity of nasal mucosa. Therefore, it is justified to perform basic allergy diagnostics in all children with AH as well as to examine the adenoids in children with AR. Nevertheless, our understanding of the complex interplay among adenoiditis, allergy and otitis media is still elusive.

Adenoidectomy is one of the most common surgical procedure in children. The most common indications for such procedure include chronic otitis media, medically refractory chronic rhinosinusitis, and airway obstruction. The nasopharyngeal space and the size of the adenoids have been evaluated using different methods of assessment, mainly X-rays, nasal flexible fiberoptic endoscopy, and direct measurements during surgery. Nasal endoscopy has now to be considered as the gold standard, being minimally invasive and allowing to identifying the etiology of nasal obstruction.

References

[1]   Eun YG, Park DC, Kim SG, Kim MG, Yeo SG. Immunoglobulins and transcription factors in adenoids of children with otitis media with effusion and chronic rhinosinusitis. *Int J Pediatr Otorhinolaryngol.* 2009; 73:1412-6.

[2]   Brandtzaeg P. Immunology of tonsils and adenoids: everything the ENT surgeon needs to know. *Int J Pediatr Otorhinolaryngol.* 2003; 67:69-76.

[3]   Casselbrant ML. What is wrong in chronic adenoiditis/tonsillitis anatomical considerations. *Int J Pediatr Otorhinolaryngol.* 1999; 49: S133-5.

[4]   Brodscy L, Koch RJ. Anatomic correlates of normal and diseased adenoids in children. *Laryngoscope.* 1992; 102:1268-74.

[5]   Fujioka M, Young LW, Girdany BR. Radiographic evaluation of adenoidal size in children: adenoidal–nasopharyngeal ratio. *AJR.* 1979; 133:401-4.

[6]   Bernstein JM, Gorfien J, Brandtzaeg P. The immunobiology of the tonsils and adenoids, in: P.L. Ogra, J. Mestecky, M.E. Lamm, W. Strober, J. Bienenstock, J.R. McGhee (Eds.), *Mucosal Immunology,* Academic, San Diego, 1999 , pp. 1339-62.

[7]   Modrzynski M, Zawisza E. An analysis of the incidence of adenoid hypertrophy in allergic children. *Int J Pediatr Otorhinolaryngol.* 2007; 71:713-9.

[8]   Carneiro-Sampaio MMS, Carbonare SB, Rozentraub RB, Araujo MNT, Ribeiro MA, Porto MHO. Frequency of selective IgA deficiency among Brazilian blood donors and healthy pregnant women. *Allergol lmmunopathol.* 1989; 17:213-6.

[9]   Kiyono H, Bienenstock J. Features of inductive and effector sites to consider in mucosal immunization and vaccine development. *Reg Immunol.* 1992; 4: 54-62.

[10] Kuper CF, Koornstra PJ, Hameleers DM, Biewenga J, Spit BJ, Duijvestijn AM, et al. The role of nasopharyngeal lymphoid tissue. *Immunol Today.* 1992; 13:219-23.

[11] Hirata CHW, Weckx LLM, Sole D, Fifueiredo CR. Serum levels of immunoglobulins in children with recurrent otitis media. *Invest Allergol Clin Immunol.* 1999; 9:106-9.

[12] Ricci A, Avanzini MA, Scaramuzza C, Castellazzi AM, Marconi M, Marseglia GL. Toll-like receptor 2-positive and Toll-like receptor 4-positive cells in adenoids of children exposed to passive smoking. *J Allergy Clin Immunol.* 2005; 115:631-2.

[13] Marseglia GL, Avanzini MA, Caimmi S, Caimmi D, Marseglia A, Valsecchi C et al. Passive exposure to smoke results in defective IFN-gamma production by adenoids in children with recurrent respiratory infections. *J Interferon & Cytokine Research.* 2009; 29:427-32.

[14] Avanzini AM, Castellazzi AM, Marconi M, Valsecchi C, Marseglia A, Ciprandi G et al. Children with recurrent otitis show defective IFN-gamma producing cells in adenoids. *Pediatr Allergy Immunol* 2008; 19: 523–526.

[15] Fireman P. Otitis media and eustachian tube dysfunction: connection to allergic rhinitis. *J Allergy Clin Immunol.* 1997; 99:S787-97.

[16] Brodsky L, Moore L, Stanievich JF, Ogra PL. The immunology of tonsils in children: The effect of bacterial load on the presence of B- and T-cell subsets. *Laryngoscope.* 1988; 98: 93-8.

[17] Brodsky L, Moore L, Stanievich J. The role of haemophilus influenzae in the pathogenesis of tonsillar hypertrophy in children. *Laryngoscope.* 1988; 98: 1055-60.

[18] Kuhn JJ, Brook I, Waters CL, Church LWP, Bianchi DA, Thompson DH. Quantitative bacteriology of tonsils removed from children with

tonsillitis hypertrophy and recurrent tonsillitis with and without hypertrophy. *Ann Otol Rhinol Laryngol.* 1995; 104: 646-52.

[19] Noble B, Gorfien J, Frankel S, Rossman J, Brodsky L. Microanatomical distribution of dendritic cells in normal tonsils. *Acta Otolaryngol.* 1996; 523: 94-7.

[20] Brodsky L, Frankel S, Gorfien J, Rossman J, Noble B. The role of dendritic cells in the development of chronic tonsillar disease in children. *Acta Otolaryngol.* 1996; 523:98-100.

[21] Kiroglu MM, Ozbilgin K, Aydogan B, Kiroglu F, Tap O, Kaya M, Ozsahinoglu C. Adenoids and Otitis Media With Effusion: A Morphological Study. *American Journal of Otolaryngology.* 1998; 19:244-50.

[22] American Academy of Pediatrics. Subcommittee on Management of Acute Otitis Media. Diagnosis and Management of Acute Otitis Media. *Pediatrics.* 2004; 113:1451-65.

[23] Saylam G, Tatar EC, Tatar I, Ozdek A, Korkmaz H. Association of Adenoid Surface Biofilm Formation and Chronic Otitis Media With Effusion. *Arch Otolaryngol Head Neck Surg.* 2010; 136:550-5.

[24] Bylander-Groth A, Stenström C. Eustachian tube function and otitis media in children. *Ear Nose Throat J.* 1998; 77:762-4, 766, 768-9.

[25] Hall-Stoodley L, Hu FZ, Gieseke A, Nistico L, Nguyen D, Hayes J, et al. Direct detection of bacterial biofilms on the middle-ear mucosa of children with chronic otitis media. *JAMA.* 2006; 296:202-11.

[26] Bluestone CD. Pathogenesis of otitis media: role of eustachian tube. *Pediatr Infect Dis J.* 1996; 15:281-91.

[27] Rosenfeld RM, Culpepper L, Doyle KJ, Grundfast KM, Hoberman A, Kenna MA, et al. Clinical practice guidelines: Otitis media with effusion. *Otolaryngol Head Neck Surg.* 2004; 130:S95-118.

[28] Hurst DS, Venge P. Evidence of eosinophil, neutrophil, and mast-cell mediators in the effusion of OME patients with and without atopy. *Allergy.* 2000; 55:435-41.

[29] Lagging E, Papatziamos G, Halldén G, Hemlin C, Härfast B, van Hage-Hamsten M. T-cell subsets in adenoids and peripheral blood related to age, otitis media with effusion and allergy. *APMIS.* 1998; 106:354-60.

[30] Marseglia GL, Poddighe D, Caimmi D, Marseglia A, Caimmi S, Ciprandi G, et al. Role of adenoids and adenoiditis in children with allergy and otitis media. *Curr Allergy Asthma Rep.* 2009; 9:460-4.

[31] Modrzynski M, Zawisza E. The influence of birch pollination on the adenoid size in children with intermittent allergic rhinitis. *Int J Pediatr Otorhinolaryngol.* 2007; 71:1017-23.

[32] Loesel LS. Detection of allergic disease in adenoid tissue. *Am J Clin Pathol.* 1984; 81:170-5.

[33] Ganzer U, Bachert C. Localization of IgE synthesis in immediate-type allergy of the upper respiratory tract. *ORL J Otorhinolaryngol Relat Spec.* 1988; 50:257-64.

[34] Fokkens WJ, Vinke JG, De Jong SS, Bogaert DPVD, Kleinjan A, Eichhorn E. Differences in cellular infiltrates in the adenoid of allergic children compared with age- and gender-matched controls. *Clin Exp Allergy* 1998; 28:187-95.

[35] Shin SY, Choi GS, Hur GY, Lee KH, Kim SW, Cho JS, et al. Local production of total IgE and specific antibodies to the house dust mite in adenoid tissue. *Pediatr Allergy Immunol.* 2009: 20:134-41.

[36] Kay AB. 'Helper' (CD4+) T cells and eosinophils in allergy and asthma. *Am Rev Respir Dis.* 1992, 145:S22–6.

[37] Godthelp T, Holm AF, Fokkens WJ Dynamics of nasal eosinophils in response to a nonnatural allergen challenge in patients with allergic rhinitis and control subjects: a biopsy and brush study. *J Allergy Clin Immunol.* 1996; 97:800–11.

[38] Woolley KL, Adelroth E, Woolley MJ Effects of allergen challenge on eosinophils, eosinophil cationic protein, and granulocyte-macrophage colony-stimulating factor in mild asthma. *Am J Respir Crit Care Med.* 1995; 151:1915–24.

[39] Bentley AM, Jacobson MR, Cumberworth V Immunohistology of the nasal mucosa in seasonal allergic rhinitis: increases in activated eosinophils and epithelial mast cells. *J Allergy Clin Immunol.* 1992; 89:877–83.

[40] Abu-Ghazaleh RJ, Fujisawa T, Mestecky J, Kyle RA, Gleich GJ. IgA-induced eosinophil degranulation. *J Immunol.* 1989: 142:2393–400.

[41] Monteiro RC, Hostoffer RW, Cooper MD, Bonner JR, Gartland GL, Kubagawa H. Definition of immunoglobulin A receptors on eosinophils and their enhanced expression in allergic individuals. *J Clin Invest.* 1993: 92:1681–5.

[42] van Nieuwkerk EB, de Wolf CJ, Kamperdijk EW, van der Baan S. Lymphoid and non-lymphoid cells in the adenoid of children with otitis media with effusion: a comparative study. *Clin Exp Immunol.* 1990; 79:233–9.

[43] Abdullah B, Hassan S, Sidek D, Jaafar H. Adenoid mast cells and their role in the pathogenesis of otitis media with effusion. *J Laryngol Otol.* 2006; 120:556-60.

[44] Wright AL, Holberg CJ, Martinez FD, Halonen M, Morgan W, Taussig LM. Epidemiology of physician-diagnosed allergic rhinitis in childhood. *Pediatrics.* 1994; 94:895-901.

[45] Huang SW, Giannoni C. The risk of adenoid hypertrophy in children with allergic rhinitis. *Ann Allergy Asthma Immunol.* 2001; 87:350-5.

[46] Ambulatory and Inpatient Procedures in the United States, National Center for Health Statistics, 1996, *http://www.cdc.gov/nchs/data/series/sr_13/sr13_139.pdf.*

[47] Brietzke SE, Brigger MT. Adenoidectomy outcomes in pediatric rhinosinusitis: A meta-analysis. *Int J Pediatr Otorhinolaryngol.* 2008; 72:1541-5.

[48] Post JC. Direct evidence of bacterial biofilms in otitis media. *Laryngoscope.* 2001; 111:2083-94.

[49] Darrow DH, Siemens C. Indications for tonsillectomy and adenoidectomy. *Laryngoscope.* 2002; 112:6-10.

[50] Coyte PC, Croxford R, McIsaac W, Feldman W, Friedberg J. The role of adjuvant adenoidectomy and tonsillectomy in the outcome of the insertion of tympanostomy tubes. *N Engl J Med.* 2001; 344:1188-95.

[51] Hammarén-Malmi S, Saxen H, Tarkkanen J, Mattila PS. Adenoidectomy does not significantly reduce the incidence of otitis media in conjunction with the insertion of tympanostomy tubes in children who are younger than 4 years: a randomized trial. *Pediatrics.* 2005; 116:185-9.

[52] National Ambulatory Medical Care Survey, National Center for Health Statistics, *http://www.cdc.gov/nchs/about/major/ahcd/ahcd1.htm.*

[53] Ramadan HH, Cost JL. Outcome of Adenoidectomy Versus Adenoidectomy With Maxillary Sinus Wash for Chronic Rhinosinusitis in Children. *Laryngoscope.* 2008; 118:871-3.

[54] Hartog B, Van Benthem PP, Prins LC, Hordijk GJ. Efficacy of sinus irrigation versus sinus irrigation followed by functional endoscopic sinus surgery. *Ann Otol Rhinol Laryngol.* 1997; 106:759-66.

[55] Rosen GM, Muckle RP, Mahowald MW, Goding GS, Ullevig C. Postoperative respiratory compromise in children with obstructive sleep apnea syndrome: can it be anticipated? *Pediatrics.* 1994; 93:784-8.

[56] Leong AC, Davis JP. Morbidity after adenotonsillectomy for paediatric obstructive sleep apnoea syndrome: waking up to a pragmatic approach. *J Laryngol Otol.* 2007; 121:809-17.

[57] Blenke EJ, Anderson AR, Raja H, Bew S, Knight LC. Obstructive sleep apnoea adenotonsillectomy in children: when to refer to a centre with a paediatric intensive care unit? *J Laryngol Otol.* 2008; 122:42-5.

[58] Isaacson G. Avoiding airway obstruction after pediatric adenotonsillectomy. *Int J Pediatr Otorhinolaryngol.* 2009; 73:803-6.

[59] Saedi B, Sadeghu M, Mojtahed M, Mahoubi H. Diagnostic efficacy of different methods in the assessment of adenoid hypertrophy. *Am J Otolaryngol.* 2010; *in press.*

[60] Yilmaz I, Caylakli F, Yilmazer C, Sener M, Ozluoglu LN. Correlation of diagnostic systems with adenoidal tissue volume: A blind prospective study. *Int J Pediatr Otorhinolaryngol.* 2008;72:1235-40.

[61] Kubba H, Bingham BJ. Endoscopy in the assessment of children with nasal obstruction, *J Laryngol Otol.* 2001; 115:380-4.

[62] Kindermann CA, Roithmann R, Lubianca Neto JF. Sensitivity and specificity of nasal flexible fiberoptic endoscopy in the diagnosis of adenoid hypertrophy in children. *Int J Pediatr Otorhinolaryngol.* 2008; 72:63-7.

[63] Ezzat WF. Role of endoscopic nasal examination in reduction of nasopharyngeal adenoid recurrence rates. *Int J Pediatr Otorhinolaryngol.* 2010; 74:404-6.

[64] Tosca MA, Riccio AM, Marseglia GL, Caligo G, Pallestrini E, Ameli F, et al. Nasal endoscopy in asthmatic children: assessment of rhinosinusitis and adenoiditis incidence, correlations with cytology and microbiology. *Clin Exp Allergy.* 2001; 31:609-15.

[65] Marseglia GL, Pagella F, Caimmi D, Caimmi S, Castellazzi AM, Poddighe D, et al. Increased risk of otitis media with effusion in allergic children presenting with adenoiditis. *Otolaryngol Head Neck Surg* 2008, 138:572-575.

[66] Marseglia GL, Pagella F, Klersy C, Barberi S, Licari A, Ciprandi G. The 10-day mark is a good way to diagnose not only acute rhinosinusitis but also adenoiditis, as confirmed by endoscopy. *Int J Pediatr Otorhinolaryngol.* 2007; 71:581-3.

In: Tonsillar Disorders
Editor: Anne C. Hallberg

ISBN: 978-1-61209-275-1
©2011 Nova Science Publishers, Inc.

Chapter II

Markers of Lymphoid Follicle Function in Chronic Tonsillitis

*Verica Avramović[1], Predrag Vlahović[*2] and Vladimir Petrović[1]*

[1]Institute of Histology and Embryology, Medical Faculty, Niš, Serbia
[2]Center for Medical Biochemistry, Clinical Center, Niš, Serbia

Abstract

The lymphoid follicle of palatine tonsil, as a B-cell-rich zone, is the site of proliferation, differentiation and selection of the antigen-stimula-ted B cells. All of these processes are taking place in specific microenvironment that is product of lymphoid follicle cells.

Methods: The microenvironment of lymphoid follicles was analyzed on tonsillar tissue specimens from patients with recurrent tonsillitis (RT) and hypertrophic tonsillitis (HT). Structural organization of lymphoid follicles was observed by scanning electron microscopy. Proliferation and differentiation of stimulated follicular B cells, as well as apoptotic and inflammatory factors in lymphoid follicles were analyzed by LSAB/HRP method on paraffin slices using monoclonal antibody for Ki-67, Bcl-2, Bax and TNF-α, respectively. The follicular immunoglobulin (Ig) -

---

* Correspondence: Predrag Vlahović, Center for Medical Biochemistry, Clinical Center Niš, Dr. Zorana Đinđića 48, 18000 Niš, Serbia, Email: predrag_vlahovic@yahoo.com

producing cells were detected by using PAP method. Moreover, we have investigated the enzyme activity of 5′-nukleotidase (5′-NT), Mg^{2+}ATPase and dipeptidyl peptidase IV (DPP IV) using enzymohistochemical and immunohistochemical methods. AgNOR method was performed to determine the cell cycle of the follicular lymphocytes. In addition to this, quantitative Image analysis of lymphoid follicles and follicular cells was also done.

Results: Both types of tonsillitis show similar distribution of Ki-67-, Bcl-2-, Bax- and TNF-α- expressing cells and Ig-producing cells as well, although number of investigated cells was different. The greater number of cells in follicular germinal centers was in G_1 phase, whereas the most of lymphocytes in mantle zone were in $S+G_2$ phase of cell cycle, with significant differences between HT and RT. Activity of 5′-NT, Mg^{2+}ATPase and DPP IV is localized in different morphological compartments of the palatine tonsil, however, each of these enzymes doesn't show the difference in localization between RT and HT.

Conclusion: The numerous factors contribute to specific environment for proliferation and differentiation of stimulated B cells in lymphoid follicles of palatine tonsil. The quantitative differences of investigated markers, used for demonstration of dynamic processes associated with follicular B cells, suggest the different immune response in tonsils with RT compared to that with HT.

Introduction

Palatine tonsil is the organ of the mucosal and systemic immune response considering recurrent upper respiratory tract infections [26, 8]. The chronic tonsillitis is the consequence of the permanent antigen stimulation during the lifetime. Two the most common forms of the chronic tonsillitis are recurrent tonsillitis (RT) and hypertrophic tonsillitis (HT).

Germinal centre (GC) of tonsillar lymphoid follicle is the site of proliferation, differentiation and clonal selection of antigen-stimulated B cells [23]. On the other hand, follicular mantle zone (MZ) is composed of memory B cells. Differentiation into plasma cells and memory B cells in GC is precisely regulated by the cellular interaction among $CD4^+$ (Th2) cells, B cells and follicular dendritic cells [9, 12, 31]. Besides this, different apoptotic factors are essentially involved in the process of B cells selection [17]. The germinal centre cells, which didn't received the signals for the positive selection, get out of their cell cycle undergoing to apoptosis [21, 16, 14]. Moreover, it is well known that numerous cytokines [1] as well as many enzymes [22] influence the differentiation and maturation of the stimulated B cells in the GC and strongly upregulate T-cell activation. In addition, some authors demonstrated that the members of tumor necrosis factor (TNF) family are crucial for B cell selection in follicular GC [24, 25].

In order to define possible differences of the functional morphology of tonsillar lymphoid follicles in RT and HT, we detected and quantified expression of biological markers of proliferation and apoptosis as well as immunological and enzymatic activity inside of lymphoid follicles.

Material and Methods

Palatine tonsils were obtained at ORL Clinic of Clinical Centre Niš, from patients aged 10 to 29 years, who had undergone elective tonsillectomy for chronic tonsillitis; 5 patients (aged 18 to 22 years) with RT and 6 patients (aged 10 to 29 years) with HT. Before the tonsillectomy, signed written consent was obtained by all patients or their parents in case of minors.

Histological preparation. After removal, each tonsil was divided into three pieces. One part was routinely processed to paraffin blocks for light microscope study. The second part was frozen on -70°C and cut in 3-5 μm thick slices for enzymohistochemical study and third part of the material was prepared for scanning electron microscope analysis.

Scanning electron microscopy. Tissue samples about 3x3x3 mm, were taken under a dissecting microscope and fixed in Zamboni's fixative at 4°C for 24 hours and transferred to 0.1 m cacodylate buffer (pH 7.2) at 4°C for further 12 hours. Samples were post fixed in 1% osmiumtetroxide for 90 minutes, placed in phosphate buffer saline for 30 minutes and dehydrated in increasing concentrations (30-100%) of ethanol. Samples were placed in ascending grades of acetone diluted in ethanol and in ascending grades of amyl acetate diluted in acetone (50-100%). Then, they were critical point dried, sputter coated with gold and examined under a JEOL JSM-5300 scanning electron microscope.

Immunohistochemistry. LSAB/HRP method was applied to define: a) proliferative activity of the lymphoid follicle cells, by using monoclonal antibody for Ki-67 antigen (dako, Denmark); b) apoptotic activity in lymphoid follicles, by using monoclonal antibodies for Bcl-2 and Bax protein (DAKO, Denmark) and c) cytokine production in lymphoid follicles, by using tumor necrosis factor alpha (TNF-α) monoclonal antibody (Santa Cruz Biotechnology, USA).

Immunohistochemistry was performed on 3 μm thick paraffin sections by using 45-minute heat-induced epitope retrieval in 0.01M citrate buffer at pH 6.0, followed by 30 minutes incubation with the primary antibody at room temperature. This was followed by staining using the DAKO LSAB/HRP kit. Streptavidin and diaminobenzidine (DAB) were added. Finally, the slides were counterstained with Mayer's hematoxylin.

Peroxidase-antiperoxidase (PAP) method [28] was performed to determined cytoplasmatic IgA, IgG and IgM in follicular B cells, on the 3 μm thick paraffin sections, using specific rabbit antihuman IgA, IgG and IgM monoclonal antibodies (DAKO, Denmark) diluted in PBS 1:2000, 1:150 and 1:1500, respectively.

Quantitative image analysis. Area and numerical areal density of lymphoid follicles and investigated follicular cells were determined by digital image analysis using Image J software. The images were obtained on microscope NU-2 (Carl Zeiss, Jena, Germany) and acquired with a web color camera MSI370i. The objective x4 was used for determination of the area and numerical areal density of lymphoid follicles, while the objective x40 was applied to determine the numerical areal density of follicular cells, i.e. the average number of cells per mm^2 of tissue. For each palatine tonsil all lymphoid follicles on the three slices were examined. For quantitative analysis of follicular cells the three slices from each palatine tonsil were used and 20 fields per slice were inspected; the distance between the slices was 30 μm. Statistical analysis of the results were performed using Mann-Whitney rank sum test.

Enzymohistochemistry. The 5′-nucleotidase (5′-NT) and Mg^{2+}ATPase were demonstrated by the method of Wachstein and Meisel [33]. Unfixed frozen sections were incubated for 45 min at 37°C in the medium containing: 0.2 M Tris-maleate buffer (pH 7.2), 2 mM lead nitrate, 1 mM magnesium chloride and 1 mM levamisole. Incubation medium contained 1mM sodium adenosine monophosphate for 5′-NT or 1mM sodium adenosine triphosphate for Mg^{2+} ATPase, used as substrates. Following incubation, sections were washed twice in distilled water, treated with fresh 1% ammonium sulphide for 2 min, rinsed in distilled water and mounted in gelatin mountant.

Detection of DPP IV (CD26) activity on frozen sections was performed according to the method of Lojda [20]. Briefly, 4mg of Gly-Pro-4-methoxy-β-naphthylamide (Sigma, Germany) was dissolved in 500 μl of *N, N*- dimethylformamide (ICN, OH). Fast blue B salt 10 mg (Gurr's, London, England) was dissolved in 9.5 ml of Dulbecco phosphate-buffered saline (PBS- pH 7.2) mixed with Gly-Pro-4-metoxy-β-naphthyl-amide solution, and the mixture was filtered through a 0.22-µm-pore-size membrane filter. The sections were incubated in this mixture for 10 min at room temperature, and the reaction was stopped by extensive washing with PBS. Serial sections were counterstained with Mayer's hematoxylin. For the negative control, the mixture was used without a substrate.

Immunohistochemical analysis of DPP IV activity was performed on the cryostat sections fixed in cold acetone at -20°C and incubated in PBS (pH 7.2) with 5% fetal calf serum for 20 min. The slides were incubated with anti/DPP IV monoclonal antibody (Bender Med System, Austria). After 1 h of incubation, the slides were incubated with fluorescein isothiocyanate-conjugated goat anti-mouse immunoglobulin (Becton Dickinson, San Jose, CA). The slides were examined under a fluorescence microscope.

Lymphocyte cell cycle. AgNOR method was used to determine the cell cycle of the follicular lymphocytes. Two paraffin sections from each tonsil were stained by AgNOR method according to Howell and Black [11]. For the 95% confidence limits and relative standard error under 0.1, 100 cells of both mantle zone and germinal center were examined on each section. The phase of the cell cycle was determined according to Alberts et al [1994] using both the number and size of AgNORs dots; cells with one large AgNOR- equavivalent to $S+G_2$ phase, cells with two or more smaller AgNORs- equavivalent to G_1, and cells without AgNOR-equavivalent to G_0 or M phase of cell cycle. The sections were examined using x100 oil-immersion objective. The differences between the groups were tested according to a two-tailed Mann-Whitney U test at rejection level of 5%.

Results

The tonsils with HT possess large lymphoid follicles where hyperplastic GC are easily distinguished from the MZ (Fig. 1a). The lymphoid follicles in tonsils with RT are smaller, and the interfollicular compartments are dominant (Fig. 1b). The mean follicle area in HT (0.38 ± 0.17 mm^2) was significantly increased compared with that in RT (0.28 ± 0.12 mm^2) (P < 0.05). Measurement of the GC area demonstrated significant differences between HT (0.26 ± 0.13 mm^2) and RT (0.17 ± 0.09 mm^2) (P < 0.01).

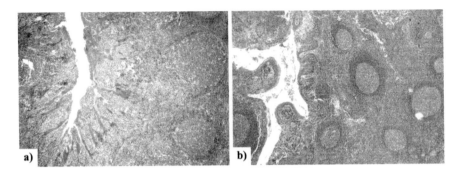

Figure 1. Light micrograph of palatine tonsil with: a) hypertrophic tonsillitis and b) recurrent tonsillitis. Observe the tonsillar crypt epithelium with pink stained stretch of keratinized parts and lymphoid follicles composed of pale-stained germinal centre and peripheral darkly-stained mantle zone. H&E. x100.

Histology of Lymphoid Follicles

Scanning electron microscopy revealed reticular cells and reticular fibers which form the framework in lymphoid follicles. There were two types of follicular reticular cells: small fibroblast-like cells (Fig. 2a) and 15-20 µm large cells with spherical protrusions and particles on their surface (Fig. 2b). Lymphocytes were present inside the follicle reticulum. The unique tonsillar crypt epithelium with openings named the micro-crypts (Fig. 2c) lay above the lymphoid tissue.

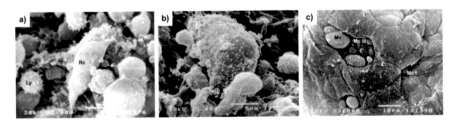

Figure 2. Scanning electron microscopy of palatine tonsil: a) Reticular fibroblast-like cells (Rc) in germinal centre form the framework; several lymphocytes (Ly) are present; next to the reticular cell there is a cell with the blebs which could be the lymphocyte in apoptosis; b) Large cell with spherical protrusions and particles on the surface possibly represents a follicular dendritic cell or macrophage; note adjacent lymphocyte; c) Tonsillar crypt epithelium show the openings – micro crypts (Mc I and Mc III) which are situated between the squamous epithelial cells with microridges; micro crypts contain large oval microvillous cells, probably antigen - presenting cells (Mv).

Proliferative and Apoptotic Activity in Lymphoid Follicles

In both studied types of tonsillitis, Bcl-2 expressing cells were found preferentially in the follicular mantle zone (Fig. 3a and 3b). Moreover, the distribution of Ki-67- positive cells was similar in RT and HT. The cells in dark zone of GC showed stronger positive reaction than the cells in GC light zone. In the follicular mantle zone, Ki-67- positive cells were scattered (Fig. 3c and 3d). Only single cells showed the clear expression of Bax. In both groups of tonsillitis, expression of Bax was presented in GC and sometime on the border between GC and mantle zone of lymphoid follicle (Fig. 3e – 3g).

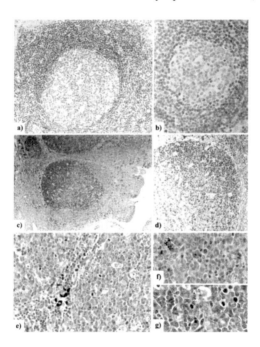

Figure 3. LSAB+/HRP method: a) Bcl-2-expressing cells are prominent in follicular mantle zone, contrary to the germinal centre which deprived from Bcl-2 expression (x200); b) detail from previous picture (x400); c) Ki-67-positive cells are dominant in the follicular germinal centres, while the scattered cells were found in mantle zone and crypt epithelium (x200); d) detail from previous picture showing part of germinal centre dark zone (x400); e) Bax is strongly expressed parafolliculary while the weak Bax-positive cells are placed in germinal centre (x400); f) Large germinal centre cells related to macrophages posses, probably, parts of phagocyted apoptotic bodies (x630); g) The cell with strongly positive reaction in cytoplasm - at the lower part of the picture (x1000).

Cytokine and Immunoglobulin Production in Lymphoid Follicles

TNF-α-producing cells were found in GC and occasionally in mantle zone of lymphoid follicles in all tonsils (Fig. 4a – 4d). Ig-producing cells were similar distibuted in tonsils with RT and HT. IgA-producing cells were associated with crypt epithelium and rarely were seen in lymphoid follicles (Fig. 4e), although IgG-producing cells were numerous beneath the crypt epithelium and a few cells were detected in GC (Fig. 4f). Predominant localization of IgM-producing cells, in a pattern of single and sparse cells, was found in CG of lymphoid follicles.

Enzymatic Activity in Lymphoid Follicles

The activity of ecto-5´-NT in both types of tonsillitis showed similar distribution. The intensive activity was presented in the lymphoid follicles, while there was no enzymatic reaction in parafollicular regions. The most intense activity of lymphoid follicles was detected in the GC, mostly in light zones (Fig. 5a). In contrast to the activity of ecto-5´-NT, a very low Mg^{2+}-ATPase activity was seen in lymphoid follicles, while the strong enzymatic reaction was found in parafollicular lymphoid tissue (Fig. 5b). The activity of DPP IV showed similar localization in tonsils with HT and RT. The strong activity was noticed in the parafollicular regions, while the GC remained unstained (Fig. 5c). On the same time, immunohystochemistry with CD26 monoclonal antibody demonstrated a weak fluorescence in GC (Fig. 5d).

Quantitative Image Analysis of Lymphoid Follicles and Follicular Cells

Table 1 shows the results obtained from the quantitative analysis of lymphoid follicles and investigated cells in tonsils with HT and RT. Numerical areal density of lymphoid follicles is higher in RT compared to that in HT.

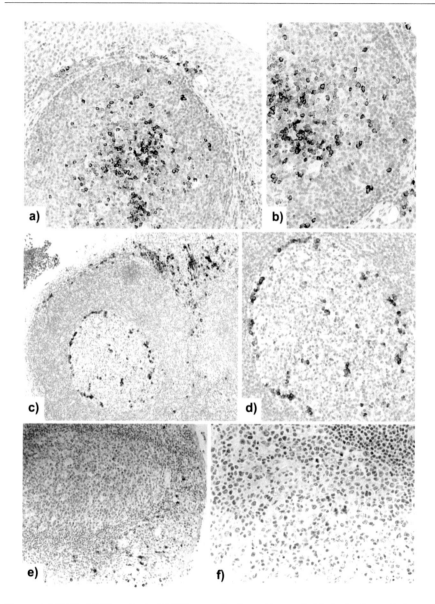

Figure 4. LSAB+/HRP method: a) TNF-α- producing cells are visible in the form of clusters in follicular germinal centre or as single cells in mantle zone in tonsils with hypertrophic tonsillitis (x400); b) detail from previous picture; c) in tonsils with recurrent tonsillitis, TNF-α- producing cells are localized on the border between germinal centre and mantle zone (x200); d) detail from previous picture (x400). PAP method: e) IgA-producing cells are numerous in crypt epithelium and a few cells are seen in germinal centre (x200); f) IgG-producing cells are seen in follicular germinal centre (x400).

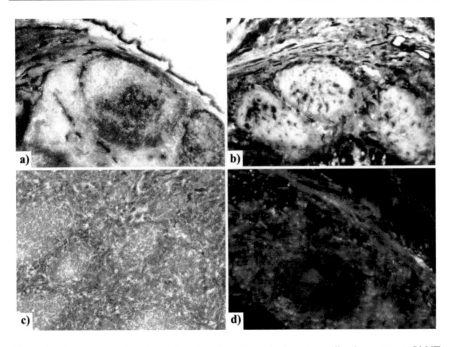

Figure 5. Enzyme activity of palatine tonsil: a) Germinal centre cells show strong 5´-NT activity; b) Mg^{2+}-ATPase activity was detected in small part of germinal centres, while the strong reaction was found in parafollicular lymphoid tissue (x200); c) DDP IV enzyme activity was presents around of lymphoid follicles and in interfollicular areas as well (x200); d) The strong immunofluorescence for CD26 was detected parafolliculary while in germinal centre of lymphoid follicles only scarce fluorescence was found (x1000).

Table 1. Number of lymphoid follicles and follicular cells per mm^2 of tonsillar slice area in hypertrophic tonsillitis (HT) and recurrent tonsillitis (RT).

Numerical areal density (N_A)	Lymphoid follicle	HT (n=6)	RT (n=5)
Lymphoid follicle	Whole	1.37 ± 0.47	1.61 ± 0.58
Ki-67 expressing cells	Dark zone	14681.45 ± 1460.47	12491.37 ± 2321.59*
	Light zone	8014.36 ± 1404.71	7844.22 ± 1360.62
	Mantle zone	1406.87 ± 393.06	1001.01 ± 540.75*
Bcl-2 expressing Cells	Mantle zone	10856.42 ± 1171.35	13253.65 ± 2226.01
	Germinal center	absent	absent
TNF-α producing cells	Whole	1517.21 ± 720.76	1260.21 ± 661.06

* - p < 0.01 vs. HT

Number of Ki-67-positive cells in lymphoid follicles was significantly different in HT and RT, concerning mantle zone (P < 0.001) and dark zone (P < 0.01) of GC. The greater number of Bcl-2-expressing cells was found in follicular mantle zone in HT, compared to that in RT, without statistical significance. Also, the number of follicular TNF-α-producing cells was greater in HT compared to RT, but this difference was not statistically significant.

Cell Cycle Analysis of Follicle Lymphocytes

The result of lymphocyte cell cycle analysis is given in Table 2, while the number and size of AgNOR dots in nuclei are shown on Figure 6.

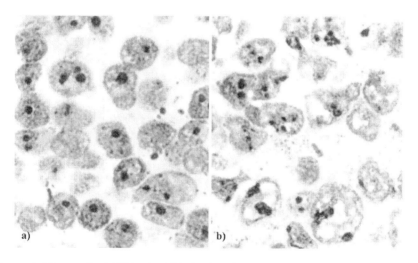

Figure 6. Silver-stained NORs in follicular lymphocytes: a) Nuclei of the mantle zone lymphocytes have, mainly, one large AgNOR; b) The numerous nuclei of germinal centre cells show two or more smaller AgNOR dots. x1250.

The greater number of germinal centre cells were in G_1 phase, compared to the cells in S+G_2 and Go+M phases. The most of lymphocytes in mantle zone were in S+G_2 phase with significant differences between HT and RT. Significant difference was found also between the mantle zone cells which are in G_1 phase.

Table 2. Number of follicle lymphocytes in different phases of cell cycle in hypertrophic (HT) and recurrent tonsillitis (RT).

Phase of cell cycle	HT (n=6)		RT (n=5)	
	Germinal centre (% of all cells)	Mantle zone (% of all cells)	Germinal centre (% of all cells)	Mantle zone (% of all cells)
G_1	79.87 ± 5.05	33.37 ± 14.23	79.66 ± 2.06	13.83 ± 5.49[*]
$S + G_2$	19.75 ± 4.98	60.00 ± 14.63	16.50 ± 2.73	79.50 ± 7.17[*]
Go + M	0.3 ± 0.74	6.62 ± 3.46	3.00 ± 3.68	6.66 ± 4.08

Data are given as means ± SD.* - p < 0.05 vs. HT

Discussion

In the present study we investigated some of numerous factors which contribute to specific microenvironment in lymphoid follicles of palatine tonsil and influence on proliferation and differentiation of antigen-stimulated B cells. The study was focused on hypertrophic tonsillitis (HT) and recurrent tonsillitis (RT), two different entity of chronic tonsillitis.

The follicles area measurement results are in agreement with those from Zhang et al [34]. Namely, mean follicle area as well as mean germinal centre area was increased in tonsils with HT compared to tonsils with RT. These results confirmed different morphological substrate in HT and RT suggesting different activity of follicular cells and, consequently, the difference in immune response in HT and RT.

Stimulated B cells inside germinal centre proliferate undergoing somatic hypermutations, selection and differentiation into memory B cells and plasma cells [8, 14]. In this study, the strong expression of biological marker of proliferative cell activity, Ki-67 in GC, confirmed previous data. We proposed that Ki-67 positive B cells of GC might be related with the localization of follicular dendritic cells (FDC). Nave [23] reported that analogous to the B cell distribution, FDC precursors are predominantly localized in the dark zone, whereas highly differentiated FDC subtypes are present in the light zone of GC.

The expression of cytokines in palatine tonsil has been examined in numerous studies [1, 9, 13, 18]. Among various cytokines, as the main pro-inflammatory cytokine of the local Th1 immune response, TNF-α was also demonstrated in tonsillar tissue. We detected TNF-α-producing cells predominantly in the light zone of GC, while there was small number of TNF-α-producing cells in mantle zone. The study of Toellner et al [31] confirmed that high percentage of germinal centre T- lymphocytes produce TNF-α in low concentrations, in contrast to the cells outside the GC, in which strong TNF-α production has been found. In our study, the most interesting was the localization of TNF-α- producing cells on the border between GC and mantle zone, suggesting the production of TNF-α from helper CD4$^+$ T cells, localized in this part of the follicle. Also, Passali et al [2004] demonstrated high TNF-α concentration in hypertrophic tonsils. Based on the mentioned findings, our result suggests the relationship of this cytokine with the distribution of Ig-producing cells, as well as the role of TNF-α in stimulation of immunoglobulin secretion.

Surjan and coworkers [30] are the first authors who quantified Ig-producing cells in tonsillar hyperplasia and chronic tonsillitis. They found a reduced number of Ig-producing cells in all morphological compartments of diseased tonsils. In our study, IgA-producing cells were localized predominantly in tonsillar crypt epithelium and subepithelialy, while IgG and IgM-producing cells were found in follicular GC. Because Ig-producing cells were scattered and rare in lymphoid follicles, we can not compare their number in RT and HT. However, our findings support the well known role of palatine tonsil in humoral immune response [7, 8, 15, 25, 26].

Lopez-Gonzales et al [21] found out that apoptotic parameters were decreased in tonsils with tonsillar hypertrophy in contrast with those of recurrent tonsillitis. Moreover, Kucera et al [16] demonstrated that proliferating and dying cells are prevalently maturing B lymphocytes undergoing clonal selection. Recently, Kondo and Yoshio [14] reported that GC cells express a large amount of Fas antigen in contrast to the lack of apoptosis inhibitor, Bcl-2. In contrast to this, mantle zone B lymphocytes expressed a high level of Bcl-2 protein and less Fas antigen.

To understand survival and death control of germinal center B cells, the expression of antiapoptotic and proapoptotic proteins, Bcl-2 and Bax, has been analyzed in lymphoid follicles. Our results demonstrated strong expression of Bcl-2 in mantle zone cells, while there was no expression of Bcl-2 protein in GC cells. This result suggests that memory B cells are preserved of apoptosis by expression of Bcl-2 protein. Contrary to this, some of GC cells expressed Bax, suggesting their death by apoptosis. Although Bcl-2 and Bax are associated with intrinsic pathway of apoptosis, no correlation between these proteins was observed in this study, what could be explained by different mechanisms of apoptosis regulation in GC cells.

In previous study we demonstrated 5'-NT and Mg^{2+}-ATPase activities in HT and RT [4]. 5'-NT associated with the cells corresponding to the light zone of germinal centers and follicular mantle zone. Besides that, in both types of tonsillitis, Mg^{2+}-ATPase activity was observed in small part of lymphoid follicles and moderate activity was seen in mantle zone. These findings suggest that the activity of these enzymes is related to B cell proliferation and differentiation into lymphoid follicles. In addition, we found significantly higher 5'-NT and Mg^{2+}-ATPase activity on isolated tonsillar mononuclear cells in HT compared to RT. Also, higher enzymes activities were obtained in isolated tonsillar mononuclear cells compared to peripheral blood mononuclear cells in patients with chronic tonsillitis [4]. These results suggest strong involvement of 5'-NT and ATPase in processes of differentiation and maturation of stimulated tonsillar B cells.

Dipeptidyl peptidase IV (DPP IV) has been investigated as a protease and as binding co-stimulatory protein. The expression of DPP IV was immuno-histochemically proven in numerous tissues and organs including lymphoid organs [10]. It has been shown that DPP IV is identical to the cell surface marker CD26 that is expressed on membrane of resting T cells, and especially on the T-cell membrane following their activation [8, 22]. Using the classical histochemical method we could not find DPP IV expression in lymphoid follicles, although immunofluorescence analysis with monoclonal antibody for CD26 demonstrated moderate fluorescence in germinal centers of some follicles [27]. We proposed that DPP IV activity correspond to the helper T cells localization, because expression of CD26 on follicular B cells is very low or absent [10]. Our observation of parafollicular DPP IV/CD26 expression in tonsils with HT and RT clearly suggests activated helper T cells in inflamed tonsils. Recently published study of DPP IV activity in serum of patients with HT and RT, before and after tonsillectomy, demonstrated significantly elevated DPP IV activity in serum of patients with HT compared to patients with RT. After tonsillectomy, enzyme activity was decreased indicating the role of DPP IV in activation of $CD4^+$ helper T cells during the permanent antigen stimulation of tonsils [32].

Berger & Berger [6] demonstrated on peripheral lymphocytes that nucleolar activity causes changes in the nucleolar size, while processes of maturation and differentiation are characterized with alterations in number of nucleoli. Since nucleolar organizer regions (NORs) are part of DNA containing genes for rRNA synthesis, the number and size of AgNORs may correlate with cell proliferation as well as with the stage of cell cycle [19]. Sugiyama et al [29], comparing cell cycle of tonsillar lymphocytes in hyperplastic and recurrent tonsillitis, found that the most lymphocytes are $S+G_2+M$ cells, compared to total tonsillar lymphocytes. This proportion was also greater in hyperplastic than in recurrent tonsillitis. Based on the size and number of AgNORs, we found that follicular lymphocytes are in different phase of cell cycle. Namely, numerous GC lymphocytes with two or more smaller nucleoli, have just started cell cycle (G_1 phase), while the mantle zone cells, with one large nucleolus - have just begun to multiply (S+G2 phase). These data demonstrate high metabolic and proliferative activity in lymphoid follicles both in HT and RT.

Conclusion

The tonsillar lymphoid follicles are very active B-cell places where the numerous factors contribute to specific environment for proliferation and differentiation of stimulated B cells. The quantitative differences in expression of proteins related to B cell proliferation, differentiation, metabolic activity and apoptosis, suggest the different immune response in tonsils with RT compared to tonsils with HT.

References

[1]   Agren, K; Brauner, A; Andersson, J. Haemophilus influenzae and streptococcus pyogenes group a challenge induce a Th1 type of cytokine response in cells obtained from tonsillar hypertrophy and recurrent tonsillitis. *ORL* 1998;60(1):35-41.

[2]   Agren, K; Lindberg, K; Samulesson, A; Blomberg, S; Forsgren, J; Rynnel-Dagöö B. What is wrong in chronic adenoiditis/tonsillitis immunological factor. *Int J Pediatr Otorhinolaryngol* 1999; 49:137-9.

[3]   Alberts, B., Bray, D., Lewis, J., Raff, M., Roberts, K., Watson, J.D. Mollecular biology of the cells. Third edition. New York; Garland Publishing; 1994;379-383.

[4]   Avramović, V; Vlahović, P; Stanković, M; Stefanović, V. Divalent cation-activated-ATPase and ecto 5'-nucleotidase activities in chronic tonsillitis. *Arch Physiol Biochem* 1998;106(2):88-90.

[5]   Avramović, V; Vlahović, P; Savić, V; Stanković, M. Localization of ecto-5'-nucleotidase and divalent cation-activated ecto-ATPase in chronic tonsillitis. *ORL* 1998;60(3):174-177.

[6]   Berger, Z; Berger J. Circadian rhythm of the lymphocyte nucleolar area. *Comp Clin Path* 2004;12:187-190.

[7]   Boyaka, PN; Wright, PF; Marinaro, M; Kiyono, H; Johnson, JE; Gonzales, RA; Ikizler, MR; Werkhaven, JA; Jackson, RJ; Fujihashi, K; Di Fabio, S; Staats, HF; McGhee, JR. Human nasopharyngeal-associated lymphoreticular tissues. Functional analysis of subepithelial and intraepithelial B and T cells from adenoids and tonsils. *Am J Pathol* 2000;157(6):2023-35.

[8]   Brandtzaeg, P. Immunology of tonsils and adenoids: everything the ENT surgeon needs to know. *Int J Pediatr Otorhinolaryngol* 2003;67(1) :s69-76.

[9]   Butch, AW; Chung, GH; Hoffmann, JW; Nahm, MH. Cytokine expression by germinal center cells. *J Immunol* 1993;150(1):39-47.

[10] Gorrell, MD; Gysbers, V; Mccaughan, GW. CD26: a multifunctional integral membrane and secreted protein of activated lymphocytes. *Scand J Immunol* 2001;54(3):249-64.

[11] Howel, WM & Black. Controlled silver-staining of nucleolus organizer regions with a protective colloidal developer: a 1. step method. *Experientia* 1980;36:1014-1015.

[12] Johansson-Lindbom, B; Ingvarsson, S; Borrebaeck, CA. Germinal centers regulate human Th2 development. *J Immunol* 2003; 171(4): 1657-66.

[13] Komorowska, A; Komorowski, J; Banasik, M; Lewkowicz, P; Tchórzewski, H. Cytokines locally produced by lymphocytes removed from the hypertrophic nasopharyngeal and palatine tonsils. *Int J Pediatr Otorhinolaryngol* 2005;69(7):937-41.

[14] Kondo, E & Yoshio, T. Expression of apoptosis regulators in germinal centers and germinal center-derived B-cell lymphomas: Insight into B-cell lymphomagenesis. *Pathol Int* 2007;57:391-397.

[15] Korsrud, FR & Brandtzaeg, P. Immune systems of human nasopharyngeal and palatine tonsils: Histomorphometry of lymphoid components and quantification of immunoglobulin-producing cells in healt and disease. *Clin Exp Immunol* 1980;39:361-370.

[16] Kucera, T; Pácová, H; Veselý, D; Astl, J; Martínek, J. Apoptosis and cell proliferation in chronic tonsillitis and oropharyngeal carcinoma: role of nitric oxide and cytokines. *Biomed Pap* 2004;148(2):225-7.

[17] Kuki, K; Hotomi, M; Yamanaka, N. A study of apoptosis in the human palatine tonsil. *Acta Otolaryngol suppl* 1996;523:68-70.

[18] Lisignoli, G; Pozzi, C; Toneguzzi, S; Tomassetti, M; Monaco, MC; Facchini, A. Different pattern of cytokine production and mRNA expression by lymphoid and non-lymphoid cells isolated from human palatine tonsil. *Int J Clin Lab Res* 1998;28(1):23-8.

[19] Lee, HJ; Lee, AH; Lee, KY; Kang, CS; Shim, SI; Kim, BK. Argyrophilic nucleolar organizer region and expression of ki-67 in malignant lymphoma. *Korean J Pathol* 2000; 34(4):257-263.

[20] Lojda, Z. Proteinases in pathology. Usefulness of histochemical methods. *J Histochem Cytochem* 1981;29:481-493.

[21] López-González, MA; Díaz, P; Delgado, F; Lucas, M. Lack of lymphoid cell apoptosis in the pathogenesis of tonsillar hypertrophy as compared to recurrent tonsillitis. *Eur J Pediatr* 1999;158(6):469-73

[22] Mentlein, R. Dipeptidyl-peptidase IV (CD26)-role in the inactivation of regulatory peptides. *Regul Pept* 1999;85(1):9-24.

[23] Nave, H; Gebert, A; Pabst, R. Morphology and immunology of the human palatine tonsil. *Anat Embryol (Berl)* 2001;204(5):367-73.

[24] Park, CS & Choi, YS. How do follicular dendritic cells interact intimately with B cells in germinal centre. *Immunology* 2005;114:2-10.

[25] Passàli, D; Damiani, V; Passàli, GC; Passàli, FM; Boccazzi, A; Bellussi, L. Structural and immunological characteristics of chronically inflamed adenotonsillar tissue in childhood. *Clin Diagn Lab Immunol* 2004;11(6):1154-7.

[26] Perry, M; Whyte, A. Immunology of the tonsils. *Immunol Today* 1998;19(9):414-21.

[27] Stankovic, M; Vlahovic, P; Avramovic, V; Todorovic, M. Distribution of dipeptidyl peptidase IV in patients with chronic tonsillitis. *Clin Vaccine Immunol* 2008;15(5):794-8.

[28] Sternberg, LA; Hardy, PH; Cuculus, JJ; Meyer, GG. The anlabeled antibody enzyme method of immunohistochemistry. *J Histochem Cytochem* 1970;18(3):315-333.

[29] Sugiyama, M; Sakashita, T; Cho, JS; Nakai, Y. Immunological and biochemical properties of tonsillar lymphocytes. *Acta Otolaryngol* (Stochk)1984;Suppl 416:45-55.

[30] Surjan, JR; Brandtzaeg, P; Berdal, P. Immunoglobulin systems in human tonsils II. Patients with chronic tonsillitis or tonsillar hyperplasia: quantification of Ig-producing cells, tonsillar morphometry and serum Ig concentrations. *Clin Exp Immunol* 1978;31:382-390.

[31] Toellner, KM; Scheel-Toellner, D; Sprenger, R; Duchrow, M; Trümper, LH; Ernst, M; Fad, HD; Gerdes, J. The human germinal centre cells, follicular dendritic cells and germinal centre T cells produce B cell-stimulating cytokines. *Cytokine* 1995;7(4):344-54.

[32] Vlahović, P; Avramović, V; Stanković, M; Savić , S; Todorović M. Elevated serum dipeptidyl peptidase IV activity in patients with chronic tonsillitis. *Ann Clin Biochem* 2007;44 (pt 1):70-4.

[33] Wachstein, M; Meisel, E. Histochemistry of hepatic phosphatases at physiological pH. *Am J Clin Pathol* 1957;27:13-23.

[34] Zhang, PC; Pang, YT; Loh, KS; Wang, DY. Comparison of histology between recurrent tonsillitis and tonsillar hypertrophy. *Clin Otolaryngol Allied Sci* 2003;28(3):235-9.

In: Tonsillar Disorders
Editor: Anne C. Hallberg

ISBN: 978-1-61209-275-1
©2011 Nova Science Publishers, Inc.

Chapter III

Ribosomal Therapy in the Prophylaxis of Recurrent Pharyngotonsillitis

Luca Guastini, Renzo Mora, Barbara Crippa,
Valentina Santomauro and Angelo Salami
ENT Department, University of Genoa, Italy

Abstract

Pharyngotonsillitis is a common illness in adults and children, often encountered by family and emergency medicine physicians. An infection in the pharynx, which is served by the lymphoid tissues of Waldeyer's ring, can spread to other parts of the ring, such as the tonsils, nasopharynx, uvula, soft palate, adenoids, and cervical lymph glands, causing pharyngitis, tonsillitis, pharyngotonsillitis, and/or rhinosinusitis. These illnesses can be acute, subacute, chronic, or recurrent.

The reasons for recurrent pharyngotonsillitis are not deeply understood yet. In the last decades several authors have tried to explain how modifications affecting the balance of a host's immunological functions on the one hand and infection agents on the other can lead to recurrent inflammatory events: although much has been written on how to manage recurrent pharyngotonsillitis, it remains a controversial topic.

The etiologic agents may be of viral or bacterial origin. Although viruses are the most common agents that cause throat infections in children, about 30% of infections are of bacterial origin. A proper treatment should provide patients with adequate coverage of aerobic as well as anaerobic pathogens so as to minimize recurrences, enhance eradication, maximize compliance and avoid resistance. Because of antibiotic resistance increase, attention has been focused on alternative treatment.

The aim of this chapter is to evaluate the efficiency of an oral ribosomal immunotherapy in the management of patients with recurrent pharyngotonsillitis.

Introduction

Pharyngotonsillitis is a common illness in adults and children, often encountered by family and emergency medicine physicians. An infection in the pharynx, which is served by the lymphoid tissues of Waldeyer's ring, can spread to other parts of the ring, such as the tonsils, nasopharynx, uvula, soft palate, adenoids, and cervical lymph glands, causing pharyngitis, tonsillitis, pharyngotonsillitis, and/or rhinosinusitis. These illnesses can be acute, subacute, chronic, or recurrent.

The most common pathogens causing pharyngotonsillitis are *group A beta-hemolytic streptococci* (GABHS), *adenovirus, Haemophilus influenzae, Haemophilus parainfluenzae, Epstein-Barr virus, and enterovirus* [1].

Although the risk of infection also depends on environmental conditions (exposure, season, geographic location) and individual variables (age, host resistance, immunity), identifying the specific underlying agent is of utmost importance for the selection of proper therapy, which assures rapid recovery and prevents complications. However, in many cases, either the culprit cannot be determined or the involvement of a potential pathogen remains uncertain.

Recent studies suggest that pharyngotonisillits may be associated with one or more interactions between GABHS, other aerobic and anaerobic bacteria, and viruses [2]. Pharyngotonisillits may be caused by viral and bacterial infections; notwithstanding, with rare exceptions only GABHS caused infections have formal indication of antibiotic treatment [3,4].

Since most acute pharyngotonisillits are caused by viruses, they do not require antibiotic treatment. In this context, it is of the utmost importance that clinicians and otolaryngologists be capable of a correct diagnosis, avoiding inappropriate antibiotic use, thus not exposing patients to unnecessary expenses, antibiotic-related risks and increase in bacterial resistance [5].

Because of antibiotic resistance increase, in the last years attention has been focused on alternative treatment. For this reason, the aim of this chapter is to evaluate the efficiency of an oral ribosomal immunotherapy in the management of patients with recurrent pharyngotonsillitis.

Clinical Presentation

In general, the onset of pharyngotonsilitis is sudden and characterized by symptoms of fever and sore throat, nausea, vomiting, headache, and rarely, abdominal pain. Physical examination at presentation reveals erythema of the throat and tonsils and enlarged cervical glands. The physician may also note an exudate or a membrane covering the tonsils, in addition to palatal petechiae, follicles, cervical adenitis, and scarlet fever rash, depending on the causative agent; none of these findings is specific [6].

The classical symptoms of viral infections, namely, cough, rhinitis, conjunctivitis, and diarrhea, are usually absent in bacterial pharyngotonsilitis. A history of exposure to the organism and presentation in winter are contributory [7].

Specifically, the clinical diagnosis of GABHS pharyngotonsillitis is based on findings of abrupt onset of fever, with or without "sore throat", in a child older than 2 years, accompanied by ill appearance, neck muscle pain, tenderness, abdominal pain, nausea, vomiting, flushed cheeks, circumoral pallor, palatal petechiae, and circular and semicircular red marks, early strawberry tongue, scarlatinaform rash, or a peculiar, sour-sweet yeasty breath odor [7].

GABHS pharyngotonsillitis tends to present with exudative pharyngitis and enterovirus pharyngotonsilits, with ulcerative lesions. *Corynebacterium diphtheriae* infection causes a bull neck and an early exudative pharynx-gotonsillitis characterized by the development of a grayish-green thick membrane that is difficult to dislodge, and when torn off, often leaves a bleeding surface. About half the patients with *Arcanobacterium hemolyticum* infection present with a scarlatiniform rash [8].

Patients with *N. gonorrhoae* pharyngotonsillitis are often asymptomatic, though some exhibit pharyngeal ulcers or exudates. Infection with anaerobic bacteria may be differentiated clinically by the presence of enlarged and ulcerated tonsils, fetid or foul odor from the mouth [8].

Besides GABHS infection, petechiae are often seen in infections due to Epstein-Barr virus, measles, and rubella viruses. Epstein-Barr virus infection is also characterized by exudative pharyngitis, liver and spleen enlargement, and cervical adenopathy; enterovirus infection by pharyngeal vesicles or ulcers and vesicles on the palms and soles in summer; herpes simplex infection by anterior oral and lip lesions and fever, and repiratory syncytial and rubella virus infections by oral erythema and Koplik spots prior to exanthema [8].

Viral pharyngotonsillitis is usually associated with nasal secretions and is generally self-limited (4-10 days), whereas bacterial illness, if left untreated, lasts longer [8].

Treatment

Primary goals of therapy for recurrent pharyngotonsillitis include preventing acute rheumatic fever and suppurative complications (eg, peritonsillar abscess). Other goals of antimicrobial therapy include improving clinical symptoms, reducing transmission, and achieving bacteriologic eradication [9].

Following an appropriate diagnosis, patients with recurrent pharynx-gotonsillitis should be treated with an antibiotic in an adequate dosage for sufficient duration to eradicate the infecting organism from the pharynx. According to several clinical practice guidelines, antibiotic therapy is indicated for patients with acute pharyngotonsillitis if the presence of GABHS has been confirmed by throat culture [9]. In order to be considered for first-line treatment of GABHS pharyngotonsillitis, the US Food and Drug Administration (FDA) requires that an antibiotic achieve an eradication rate of at least 85% in a statistically adequate and well-controlled multicenter trial, in which bacteriologic eradication correlates with clinical cure [9].

In selecting antibiotic therapy, it is important to consider the efficacy, safety, antimicrobial spectrum, dosing schedule, likely compliance with therapy, and cost.

Several classes of antibiotics have been evaluated in clinical studies of the treatment of recurrent pharyngotonsillitis, including the penicillins, cephalosporins, macrolides, ketolides, and clindamycin [9]. *Both the American Academy of Pediatrics (AAP) and Infectious Diseases Society of America guidelines (IDSA) list penicillin as the agent of choice for first-line treatment of GABHS pharyngotonsillitis due to its proven efficacy, safety, narrow spectrum, and low cost [9]. For young children, amoxicillin may be preferred to penicillin, since the suspension is more palatable.* For patients unlikely to complete the full 10-day course of oral antibiotic therapy, an intramuscular injection of benzathine penicillin G is preferred.

According to the recent IDSA guidelines, erythromycin is identified as a suitable alternative for patients allergic to penicillin; first-generation cephalosporins are also recommended, providing the patient does not have immediate-type hypersensitivity to b-lactam antibiotics [9]. Cephalosporins and macrolides have demonstrated greater bacteriologic eradication and clinical resolution of infection compared with penicillins [10-12].

The 2006-2007 Nelson's Pocket Book of Pediatric Antimicrobial Therapy recommends cephalosporins as first-line treatment, representing what may be a justified challenge to AAP and IDSA guidelines that recommend penicillin as the preferred first-line therapy, with other antibiotics reserved for recurrences or treatment failures [13].

Lack of bacteriologic eradication can lead to lost school days for the child, lost workdays for parents, and transmission of infection to siblings and playmates, as well as increased treatment failure and recurrence. Indeed, treatment failure rates with penicillin have increased since the early 1970s, when the bacteriologic failure rate after 10 days of penicillin therapy was approximately 2% to 10%. Several recent studies suggest that treatment failure after penicillin therapy may now approach 25% to 35% in the United States [14].

Despite the rising incidence of penicillin resistance, there has not been an overwhelming increase in the incidence of acute rheumatic fever. While the incidence and severity of acute rheumatic fever in the United States has declined significantly over the past five decades, reports beginning in the mid 1980s have cited a resurgence of this complication in several areas of the country [15-17].

Although the current incidence of acute rheumatic fever is still significantly lower than during the pre-antibiotic era, it still warrants consideration by physicians treating pediatric patients presenting with pharyngotonsillitis.

The pharynx may be co-colonized by bacterial pathogens that can inactivate penicillins and make them ineffective against GABHS. Copathogenicity in acute GABHS pharyngotonsillitis may occur when b-lactamaseproducing strains of *Haemophilus influenzae, Haemophilus parainfluenzae, Moraxella catarrhalis*, or *Staphylococcus aureus* colonize the inflamed pharynx [14]. Although these organisms are generally not pathogenic in the pharynx, they can produce the enzyme b-lactamase, which inactivates penicillins that are not b-lactamase-stable.

A clear association has been established in the therapy of GABHS pharyngotonsillitis between the failure of patients to respond to penicillin and the preexistence of b-lactamase-producing bacteria (BLPB) in their pharyngo-tonsillar flora [11]. More than 75% of tonsils were removed because of recurrent tonsillitis harboring BLPB [18]. Free b-lactamase was detected in the core of most of those tonsils. Antibiotics that are effective against GABHS and are also resistant to b-lactamase, such as cefuroxime axetil, cefdinir, or cefpodoxime, attain higher success eradication rates in relapsing GABHS pharyngotonsillitis [18].

Penicillin failure may also be caused by the eradication of normally protective flora, particularly a-hemolytic streptococci (AHS). AHS protect the pharynx from GABHS colonization by producing antibiotic-like substances called *bacteriocins* that inhibit GABHS growth as well as other growth-inhibitory substances [19]. AHS may also suppress GABHS growth by utilizing the nutrients in the nasopharyngeal environment essential for GABHS colonization. Penicillin is known to potently suppress AHS, which may then impair its protective properties. Patients who have recolonization with AHS after a course of antibiotic therapy have been shown to be less likely to develop recurrent GABHS pharyngitis than those without recolonization [20].

Missing doses or, particularly in twice-daily dosing regimens, not receiving the full dosage can be expected to reduce the effectiveness of antibiotic therapy. Penicillin V has a short half-life and administering it only twice daily may lead to a greater rate of failures. Amoxicillin once or twice daily may lead to better compliance while maintaining efficacy, and this approach warrants further study to explore microbiological outcomes [14].

These evidences highlight as the reasons for recurrent pharyngotonsillitis are not deeply understood yet. The pharynx of children and adults has a resident microbial flora which usually does not harm the subjects but constitutes a reservoir of pathogens implicated in the upper respiratory tract infections. In the last decades several authors have tried to explain how modifications affecting the balance of a host's immnological functions on the one hand and infection agents on the other can lead to recurrent inflammatory events: it has been stated that the viral and/or bacterial infection leads to a shift from a resident flora of commensals to one of more numerous and various pathogens [21].

At present, patients affected by recurrent pharyngotonsillitis are cured by means of antibacterial and symptomatic therapy. As for paediatric patients, antibacterial therapy is still the traditional approach. Because of antibiotic resistance increase, attention has been focused on the possibility of vaccinating patients against the responsible pathogens.

For these reasons, the aim of this chapter is to report our experience with an oral ribosomal immunotherapy in the prophylaxis of recurrent pharynx-gotonsillitis affecting children and adults.

Personal Experiences

Patients aged more than 4 years old with recurrent pharyngotonsillitis (at least three acute episodes of tonsillitis in the last year) were treated with ribosomal therapy: patients underwent ribosomal prophylaxis with Immucytal (1 tablet daily, 8 days a month for 3 months). At the beginning, at the end and 6 months after start, all patients underwent medical history, ENT examination, plasma levels of immunoglobulins class G, A, M (IgG, IgA, IgM), pharyngeal swabbing (with and without tonsillar squeezing) and subjective assessment of symptoms by patients' parents on the basis of a 0—4 scale (much better—much worse).

Frequency, duration, severity and social impact of pharyngotonsillitis episodes were also adopted as valid criteria. At each control the following parameters were checked: number of episodes (1, 2 or >2), duration (<3/3—6/>6 days), fever (yes/no), medical consultation (yes/no), disease frequency (once/twice/>twice per month), ancillary therapy (none/symptomatic only/antibacterials).

Serum concentration of immunoglobulins of class G and A were significantly ($p<0.05$) higher when measured after 3 months and 6 months after start. There was a moderate increase of IgM titers, which, nonetheless, did not reach statistical significance.

With regard to pharyngeal swabbing, incomplete eradication or re-infection was recorded in 18% of patients treated 6 months after start.

At the end of the study, each patient treated with ribosomal therapy presented a subjective decrease of symptoms. The mean value on the subjective evaluation scale fell from 3.8 before the treatment to 1.8 after it.

The patients treated with the ribosomal therapy experienced a significant improvement of some clinical parameters. From the second visit (i.e. at the end of the therapy) the reduction of the infection episodes proved to be significant. At the end, a significant improvement ($p<0.05$) was also observed as far as the incidence of fever, duration of episodes ($p<0.05$) and ancillary therapy ($p< 0.05$). No patient experienced side effects from the treatment.

Discussion

Anaerobes (Peptostreptococci and Bacteroides species) are the chief components of the normal human oropharyngeal flora and are the main cause of bacterial infections of the upper respiratory tract. They are isolated together with aerobic organisms, generally (beta-haemolytic group A Streptococci, *Streptococcus pyogenes*, *Streptococcus pneumoniae*, *Haemophilus influenzae* and *Moraxella catarrhalis*) [21-24]. Therapy should provide for adequate coverage of aerobic and anaerobic pathogens in order to minimize recurrences, enhance eradication, maximize compliance and avoid creating resistance.

The treatment or prophylaxis of upper respiratory tract infections with penicillins can generate bacterial resistance caused by the production of beta-lactamase or changes in the penicillin-binding proteins. Therapeutic use of antimicrobial agents that preserve the normal flora but overcome penicillin-susceptible or -resistant pathogens may enhance recovery from upper respiratory tract infections. There is some evidence that penicillin therapy is less satisfactory than in former years. Several explanations have been suggested, including inadequate pharmacokinetic properties, poor patient compliance, penicillin tolerance, re-infection and carrier state, and co-pathogen colonization with, for example, *Staphylococcus aureus*, *H. influe-nzae* or *M. catarrhalis*, which produce beta-lactamase, thereby deactivating penicillin before it can exert any effect.

Recurrent pharyngotonsillitis is a common infection and for some individuals constitutes a great problem owing to frequent recurrence. Despite its high incidence and numerous studies, the pathogenesis of recurrent pharyngotonsillitis is not fully understood. Tonsils and adenoids are respon-sible for regional immune effector and inductor functions. The epithelial surface is a site for bacterial attachment and is covered by a viscous secretion known to bind the microorganisms, but also to contain locally produced immunoglobulins. From the surface deep crypts penetrate into the tissue and are outlined by a specialized epithelium with dendritic cells and macrophages: a common hypothesis is that the pathogenic bacteria, after adherence to the tonsillar epithelium, invade the parenchyma and thereby establish the infection. The prevalence of potential respiratory pathogens on the tonsillar surface of patients with moderate symptoms of recurrent pharyngotonsillitis and/or tonsillar hypertrophy differs only slightly from that of patients without symptoms of adenotonsillar disease. Therefore, variations in the microbial flora do not seem to play an essential role in patients who have a predisposition to tonsillar disease [21].

At present, the cure of pharyngotonsillitis is based on antibacterial and symptomatic therapy. It is difficult to develop an appropriate antibiotic treatment for patients with recurrent pharyngotonsillitis because of the limitations of traditional tonsillar microflora sampling and because of the increasing incidence of beta-lactamase producing bacteria. Another problem is that in the human host, the bacterial pathogens may exist as a community of bacteria surrounded by a glycocalyx (biofilm) that is adherent to the mucosal surface with impaired host defense. Biofilms generate planktonic, nonadherent bacterial forms that may metastasize infection and generate systemic illness: if not deeply invading, most bacteria involved in this process are either covered by a thick inflammatory infiltrate or located within macrophages; this distribution of the bacteria within adenoids may be responsible for the failure of antibiotic therapy.

A purulent process can persist during asymptomatic pharyngotonsillitis. If not deeply invading, most bacteria involved in this process are either covered by a thick inflammatory infiltrate or located within macrophages. The distribution of the bacteria within tonsils may be responsible for the failure of antibiotic therapy.

With the emergence of resistant strains and the change in the distribution of pharyngotonsillitis bacteria over the time, preventive strategies such as ribosomal immunotherapy may represent a valid alternative approach [21-24].

Several studies demonstrated that immunoglobulins influence the colonization of pharynx bacteria and highlighted their inhibitory effects against pharyngeal colonization.

Bacterial ribosomes have been widely used as immunostimulants, in the prevention of upper respiratory tract infections. These subcellular structures are suspected to act as antigen carriers, and to trigger specific immune responses in mucosae associated lymphoid tissues (MALT).

Ribosomes are the components of cells that make proteins from amino. The word ribosome comes from ribonucleic acid and the Greek: soma (meaning body) Ribosomes are made from complexes of RNAs and proteins. Ribosomes are divided into two subunits, one larger than the other. The smaller subunit binds to the mRNA, while the larger subunit binds to the tRNA and the amino acids. When a ribosome finishes reading a mRNA, these two subunits split apart. Ribosomes have been classified as ribozymes, since the ribosomal RNA seems to be most important for the peptidyl transferase activity that links amino acids together [25].

Ribosomes from bacteria have significantly different structure and RNA sequences. These differences in structure allow some antibiotics to kill bacteria by inhibiting their ribosomes, while leaving human ribosomes unaffected. The ribosomes in the mitochondria of eukaryotic cells resemble those in bacteria, reflecting the evolutionary origin of this organelle [25].

Immucytal contains both proteoglycans deriving from K. pneumoniae and ribosomes deriving from four different bacterial strains (i.e. K. pneumoniae, Streptococcus pneumoniae, H. influenzae, Streptococcus pyogenes A) [21-24].

The active components of Immucytal act locally through direct contact with lymphoid tissue associated to intestinal mucous. The oral immunization determines a clonal expansion of antigen-specific lymphocytes, both in the lymphoid tissue associated to intestinal mucous and in the peripheral blood. It is also able to determinate a selective homing in the lymphoid tissue associated to bronchial mucous. In particular, the specific B-cell response is correlated with a high level of seric immunoglobulins, while the specific T-cell response is correlated with a high level of CD4 and CD8 lymphocytes [21-24].

The only possible side effects of Immucytal are rhinorrhea and some transient subfebrile episodes while it proved to have no interaction whatsoever with other drugs.

Because of its proteoglycans and ribosomes from common bacterial strains, Immucytal has specific immunostimulant properties. It can stimulate both non-specific immune response and specific antibody production. It can stimulate the activity of macrophages, polymorphonuclear cells and natural killer cells in leukocytes isolated in human peripheral blood. It can also modulate polymorphonuclear leukocytes when administered alone or in association with antibacterials [21-24].

For these reasons, ribosomal immunotherapy enhances both specific and non-specific immunity against the most common pathogens involved in pharyngotonsillitis [21-24].

The stimulation of the specific (adaptive) immune response, related to the activation of dendritic cells, allows Th-1 polarization with a consequent reduced Th2 response by the production of interleukin (IL) 12 [24]. IL-12 is a signal that helps send native CD4 T cells towards a Th1 phenotype [24]. These findings explain the significant decreased IgE levels in the patients treated with ribosomal therapy.

Past experiment showed that proteoglycans are able to induce the production of transforming growth factor beta (TGF-b) from human B-lymphocytes, suggesting that this cytokine could induce the immunoglobulin switch from IgM to IgA in the mucosal tissue after oral administration of ribosomal immunotherapy. These observations justify the not increased IgM levels observed in the patients treated with ribosomal therapy [24].

The significant increase of serum A-immunoglobulins highlights the therapeutic effectiveness of this approach for the treatment of patients affected by recurrent pharyngotonsillitis [21-24].

In the last year, several studies have demonstrated the immunostimulant activity of various bacterial extracts which seem to target not only the bacteria from which such extracts are made of, but also other pathogens responsible for the most common infections by means of non-specific mechanisms [21-24].

The positive effects of Immucytal lasted until the end of the 6-month period. The oral immunization seems to generate a rapid and long-lasting immune response, building up memory cells. These cells, in turn, seem to stimulate the pharyngeal lymphoid tissue response against potential pathogens or stronger ribosomal preparations.

The significant changes of serum immunoglobulins highlight the therapeutic effectiveness of this approach: the positive effects of ribosomal therapy lasted until the end of the 6-month period. The oral immunization seems to generate a rapid and long-lasting immune response, building up memory cells. These cells, in turn, seem to stimulate the Waldeyer's ring response against potential pathogens or stronger ribosomal preparations.

The active components of Immucytal act locally through direct contact with lymphoid tissue: the oral immunization determines a clonal expansion of antigen-specific lymphocytes, both in the lymphoid tissue associated to intestinal mucous and in the peripheral blood. It is also able to determinate a selective homing in the lymphoid tissue associated to bronchial mucous. In particular, the specific B-cell response is correlated with a high level of seric immunoglobulins, while the specific T-cell response is correlated with a high level of CD4 and CD8 lymphocytes [24].

Moreover, the weak impact of its collateral effects suggests the possibility to repeat the trial in order to strengthen the effectiveness of the drug [21-24].

Conclusions

The airways are the main gateway to environmental pathogens. The mucous membrane carpeting them is a natural barrier equipped with highly efficient biochemical, mechanical and immunological defence systems. The immune defences of the nasal cavities are part of the mucosal associated lymphoid tissue (MALT), which comprises in particular Waldeyer's ring as an effector and informative system. Secretory IgA is the main humoral effector. Both systems appear to play a fundamental role in providing host protection [26].

If tissue defences become ineffective inflammation and infection result. Persistence of infection can be complicated by sinusitis, otitis, laryngitis and bronchitis. Although viruses are usually the primary cause of pathology, superinfections with bacteria are frequent [21-24].

Although the usual expression of pharyngotonsillitis can be mild, its recurrent nature may make it disabilitating and generate therapeutic difficulties. The frequency of these recurrences may also be indicative of inadequate immune protection, suggesting that immunostimulant treatment might be effective in reducing the frequency of these recurrences [27].

On the basis of the data gathered, it is possible to affirm that ribosomal therapy is a suitable option for the treatment of patients with recurrent pharyngotonsillitis. *A short treatment with ribosomal therapy proved to be effective both in terms of clinical* (with a decrease in the number of acute episodes of pharyngotonsillitis) *and bacteriological effects* (with significant eradication of Streptococcus beta-haemoliticus from the pharynx).

References

[1] Serra, A.; Schito, G.C.; Nicoletti, G.; Fadda. G. A therapeutic approach in the treatment *Int J* Immunopathol Pharmacol, 2007, 20, 607-17.

[2] Brook, I. The role of anaerobic bacteria in tonsillitis. *Int J Pediatr Otorhinolaryngol*, 2005; 69, 9-19.

[3] Poisson, R; Meier, FA; Johnson, J. Effects of a Rapid Antigen Test For Group A Streptococcal Pharyngitis on Physician Prescribing and Antibiotic Costs. *Arch Intern Med,* 1990, 150, 1696-700.

[4]   Kaplan, EL. The Rapid Identification of Group A Beta Hemolytic Streptococci in Upper Respiratory Tract. *Pediatrics Clinics of North America,* 1988, 35, 535-42.

[5]   Brook, I. Antibacterial Therapy for Acute Group A Streptococcal Pharyngotonsillitis: Short-Course versus Traditional 10-Day Oral Regimens. *Pediatrics Drugs,* 2002, 4, 747-54.

[6]   Motta, G; Esposito, E; Motta, S; Mansi, N; Cappello, V; Cassiano, B; Motta, G Jr. The treatment of acute recurrent pharyngotonsillitis. *Acta Otorhinolaryngol Ital,* 2006, 26, 5-29.

[7]   Salami, A; Delle piane, M; Crippa, B; Mora, F; Guastino, L; Jankowska, B; Mora, R. Sulphurous water *Int J Pediatr Otorhinolaryngol,* 2008, 72, 1717-22.

[8]   Brook, I. Current management *Eur Arch Otorhinolaryngol,* 2009, 266, 315-23.

[9]   Bisno, AL; Gerber, MA; Gwaltney, JM Jr; Kaplan, EL; Schwartz, RH. Practice guidelines for the diagnosis and management of group A streptococcal pharyngitis. *Clin Infect Dis,* 2002, 35, 113-125.

[10] Brook, I. Failure of penicillin to eradicate group A b-hemolytic streptococci tonsillitis: causes and management. *J Otolaryngol,* 2001, 30, 324-329.

[11] Brook, I. The role of b-lactamase-producing bacteria in the persistence of streptococcal tonsillar infection. *Rev Infect Dis,* 1984, 6, 601-607.

[12] Brook, I. & Hirokawa, R. (1985). Treatment of patients with a history of recurrent tonsillitis due to group A b-hemolytic streptococci. A prospective randomized study comparing penicillin, erythromycin, and clindamycin. *Clin Pediatr,* 24, 331-336.

[13] Bradley, J.S., & Nelson, J.D. (2006). *Nelson's Pocket Book of Pediatric Antimicrobial Therapy* (16th ed). Miami, AWWE Medical Publishers.

[14] Pichichero, ME; Casey, JR; Mayes, T; Francis, AB; Marsocci, SM; Murphy, AM; Hoeger, W. Penicillin failure in streptococcal tonsillopharyngitis:causes and remedies. *Pediatr Infect Dis J,* 2000, 19, 917-923.

[15] Lee, G.M. & Wessels, M.R. (2006). Changing epidemiology of acute rheumatic fever in the United States. *Clin Infect Dis,* 42, 448-450.

[16] Wolfe, RR. Incidence of acute rheumatic fever: a persistent dilemma. *Pediatrics,* 2000, 105, 1375.

[17] Kavey, R.E. & Kaplan, E.L. (1989). Resurgence of acute rheumatic fever. *Pediatrics,* 84, 585-586.

[18] Brook, I. Role of b-lactamase-producing bacteria in the failure of penicillin to eradicate group A streptococci. *Pediatr Infect Dis*, 1985, 4, 491-495.

[19] Brook, I. The role of bacterial interference in otitis, sinusitis and tonsillitis. *Otolaryngol Head Neck Surg,* 2005, 133, 139-146.

[20] Roos, K; Holm, SE; Grahn-Hakansson, E; Lagergren, L. Recolonization with selected alpha-streptococci for prophylaxis of recurrent streptococcal pharyngotonsillitis—a randomized placebo-controlled multicentre study. *Scand J Infect Dis*, 1996, 28, 459-462.

[21] Mora, R; Dellepiane, M; Crippa, B; Salami, A. Ribosomal therapy *Int J Pediatr Otorhinolaryngol*, 2007, 71, 257-61.

[22] Mora, R; Barbieri, M; Passali, GC; Sovatzis, A; Mora, F; Cordone, MP. A preventive measure for otitis media in children with upper respiratory tract infections. *Int J Pediatr Otorhinolaryngol,* 2002, 63, 111-118.

[23] Mora, R; Ralli, G; Passali, FM; Crippa, B; Ottoboni, S; Mora, F; Barbieri, M. Short ribosomal prophylaxis in the prevention of clinical recurrence of chronic otitis media in children. *Int J Pediatr Otorhinolaryngol*, 2004, 68, 83-89.

[24] Mora, R; Dellepiane, M; Crippa, B; Guastini, L; Santomauro, V; Salami, A. Ribosomal therapy in the treatment of recurrent acute adenoiditis. *Eur Arch Otorhinolaryngol*, 2010, 267, 1313–1318.

[25] Benne, R. & Sloof, P. (1987). Evolution of the mitochondrial protein synthetic machinery. *BioSystems*, 21, 51–68.

[26] McGhee, JR; Mestecky, J; Dertzbaugh, MT; Eldridge, JH; Hirasawa, M; Kiyono, H. The mucosal immune system: from fundamental concepts to vaccine development. *Vaccine*, 1992, 10, 75-88.

[27] Lambert-Zechovsky, N; Bingen, E; Salord, JC; Proux, ML. Epiddmiologie des infections ORL et broncho-pulmonaires. Etude de 221 germes dans 202 prélèvements. *Gaz Med*, 1984, 91, 11-15.

In: Tonsillar Disorders
Editor: Anne C. Hallberg

ISBN: 978-1-61209-275-1
©2011 Nova Science Publishers, Inc.

Chapter IV

Tonsillar Disorders: Etiology, Diagnosis and Treatment

Chen-feng Qi, Herbert C. Morse III and
Shao Xiang
Laboratory of Immunopathology, NIAID, NIH
Rockville, Maryland, USA

Abstract

The tonsils, located at the back of the throat, are part of Waldeyer's ring located in the pharynx and the back of the oral cavity. They are considered part of the immune system, which is the primary line of defense against infection by bacteria and viruses. Tonsillar diseases and conditions include infection, cancer, hypertrophied tonsils and "kissing tonsils", and both acute and chronic tonsillar infections are very common in children. This review discusses the causes of various tonsillar diseases and conditions along with their treatments and will also include primary tonsillar infections leading to other morbidities. For example, some tonsillar infections are associated with rheumatic joint and heart conditions. Furthermore, because of the importance of tonsillar function in the overall immune system, the indications for and effects of tonsillectomy will be reviewed.

Structure and Function of Tonsils

The palatine tonsil is one of the mucosa-associated lymphoid tissues (MALT), located at the entrance to the upper respiratory and gastrointestinal tracts to protect the body from the entry of exogenous material through mucosal sites. Consequently, it is a site of and potential focus for infections, and is one of the chief immunocompetent tissues in the oropharynx. It forms part of the Waldeyer's ring, which comprises the nasopharyngeal tonsil or adenoid (NT), the paired tubal tonsils (TT), the paired palatine tonsils (PT) and the lingual tonsil (LT).

In children, the tonsils are common sites of infections that may give rise to acute or chronic tonsillitis. However, it is still an open question whether tonsillar hypertrophy is also caused by persistent infections. Tonsillectomy is one of the most common major operations performed on children. The indications for the operation have been complicated by controversy over the benefits of removing a chronically infected tissue and the possible harm caused by eliminating an important immune responsive tissue.

The information that is necessary to make a rational decision to resolve this controversy can be obtained by understanding the immunological potential of the normal palatine tonsils and comparing these functions with the changes that occur in the chronically diseased counterparts.

Stratified epithelium (e) covers the surface of the throat and continues as a lining of the crypt. Beneath this surface are numerous nodules (f) of lymphoid tissue. Many lymph cells (dark-colored region) pass from the nodules toward the surface and will eventually mix with the saliva as salivary corpuscles (s).

Palatine tonsils consist of an extensive system of crypts, which result in a large internal surface. The tonsils contain four lymphoid compartments that influence immune functions, namely the reticular crypt epithelium, the extrafollicular area, the mantle zones of lymphoid follicles, and the follicular germinal centers. In human palatine tonsils, the very first part exposed to the outside environment is tonsillar epithelium.

The human palatine tonsils (PT) are covered by stratified squamous epithelium that extends into deep and partly branched crypts, which number about 10 to 30. The crypts greatly increase the contact surface between environmental influences and lymphoid tissue. In an average adult palatine tonsil, the estimated epithelial surface area of the crypts is 295 cm^2, in addition to the 45 cm^2 of epithelium covering the oropharyngeal surface.

The crypts extend through the full thickness of the tonsil reaching almost to its hemicapsule. In healthy tonsils, the openings of the crypts are fissure-like, and the walls of the lumina are in apposition. A computerized three-dimensional reconstruction of the palatine tonsil crypt system showed that in the centre of the palatine tonsil are tightly packed ramified crypts that join with each other, while on the periphery there is a rather simple and sparse arrangement.

The crypt system is not merely a group of invaginations of the tonsillar epithelium but a highly complicated network of canals with special types of epithelium and with various structures surrounding the canals, such as blood and lymphatic vessels and germinal centers.

Macrophages and other white blood cells also concentrate in tonsillar crypts in response to the microorganisms that are attracted to the crypts. Accordingly, the tonsillar crypts serve a forward sentry role for the immune system, by providing early exposure of immune system cells to infectious organisms which may be introduced into the body via food or other ingested matter.

Cytokines are humoral immunomodulatory proteins or glycoproteins which control or modulate the activities of target cells, resulting in gene activation and thereby leading to mitotic division, growth and differentiation, migration, or apoptosis. Cytokines are produced by a wide range of cell types upon antigen-specific and non-antigen specific stimuli. It has been reported by many studies that the clinical outcome of many infectious, autoimmune, and malignant diseases appears to be influenced by the overall balance of production (profiles) of pro-inflammatory and anti-inflammatory cytokines. Therefore, determination of cytokine profiles in tonsils will provide key information for further in-depth analysis of the causes and underlying mechanisms of these disorders, as well as the roles and possible interactions between T- and B-lymphocytes and other immunocompetent cells.

The cytokine network represents a very sophisticated and versatile regulatory system that is essential to the immune system for overcoming the various defense strategies of microorganisms. Several studies have shown that T helper type 1 (Th1) and Th2 cytokines and cytokine mRNA are both detectable in Tonsillar Hypertrophy (TH) and Recurrent Tonsillitis (RT) groups. They showed that the human palatine tonsil is an active immunological organ containing a wide range of cytokine-producing cells. Both Th1 and Th2 cells are involved in the pathophysiology of TH and RT conditions. Indeed, human tonsils persistently harbor microbial antigens, even when the subject is asymptomatic of ongoing infection. It could also be an effect of ontogeny of the immune system.

However, the tonsillar crypts often provide such an inviting environment to bacteria that bacterial colonies may form solidified "plugs" or "stones" within the crypts. In particular, sufferers of chronic sinusitis or post-nasal drip frequently suffer from these overgrowths of bacteria in the tonsillar crypts. These small whitish plugs, termed "tonsilloliths" and sometimes known as "tonsil stones," have a foul smell and can contribute to bad breath; furthermore, they can obstruct the normal flow of pus from the crypts, and may irritate the throat (people with tonsil stones may complain of the feeling that something is stuck in their throat).

Tonsil Diseases

Acute Tonsillitis

A bacteria or virus infects the tonsils, causing swelling and a sore throat. The tonsil may develop a gray or white coating (exudate). When infected with *Streptococci*, numerous small yellowish-white plaques (white spots) appear in the crevices (tonsilar crypts) that are visible over the surfaces of the tonsils. Tonsillitis is common, especially in children. The condition can occur occasionally or recur frequently.

Etiology
Streptococci are the most common cause of acute tonsillitis. *Streptococcus* is a genus of spherical Gram-positive bacteria. One species of *Streptococcus*, *Streptococcus pyogenes,* is the cause of Group A streptococcal infections, including tonsillitis. If the infection is not treated, this bacterium can also cause disease in the form of post-infectious "non-pyogenic" (not associated with local bacterial multiplication and pus formation) syndromes. These autoimmune-mediated complications follow a small percentage of infections and include rheumatic fever and acute post-infectious glomerulonephritis. Both conditions appear several weeks following the initial streptococcal infection. Rheumatic fever is characterized by inflammation of the joints and/or heart following an episode of Streptococcal pharyngitis.

Adenoviruses are medium-sized (90–100 nm), nonenveloped (naked) icosahedral viruses composed of a nucleocapsid and a double-stranded linear

DNA genome. Adenoviruses were first isolated in human adenoids, from which the name is derived. Adenovirus infections most commonly cause illnesses of the respiratory system; however, depending on the infecting serotype, they may also cause various other illnesses, such as gastroenteritis, conjunctivitis, cystitis, and rashes.

Other virus also can be related with acuter tonsillitis and these include influenza virus, Epstein-Barr virus, parainfluenza viruses, enteroviruses, and herpes simplex virus. Because there is no virus-specific therapy, serious viral illness can be managed only by treating symptoms and complications of the infection.

Diagnosis and Tonsil Tests

An acute tonsillitis is usually diagnosed based on history and physical examination. The main symptoms of tonsillitis are inflammation and swelling of the tonsils, sometimes severe enough to block the airways. Other symptoms include:

- Throat pain or tenderness
- Redness of the tonsils
- A white or yellow coating on the tonsils
- Painful blisters or ulcers on the throat
- Hoarseness or loss of voice
- Headache
- Loss of appetite
- Ear pain
- Difficulty swallowing or breathing through the mouth
- Swollen glands in the neck or jaw area
- Fever, chills
- Bad breath

In children, symptoms may also include:
- Nausea
- Vomiting
- Abdominal pain

Diagnostic Tests

- Throat (pharynx) swab: A doctor rubs a cotton swab on the tonsils and throat and sends the swab for tests. Usually this is done to check for bacteria such as *Streptococcus*.
- Monospot test: A blood test can detect certain antibodies, which can help confirm that a person's symptoms are due to mononucleosis.
- Epstein-Barr virus antibodies: If a monospot test is negative, antibodies in the blood against EBV might help diagnose mononucleosis.

When acute tonsillitis occurs frequently, it may turn into recurrent tonsillitis. Recurrent infection has been variably defined as from four to seven episodes of acute tonsillitis in one year, five episodes for two consecutive years or three episodes per year for 3 consecutive years.

Treatment

Treatment for tonsillitis will depend in part on the cause. To determine the cause, a rapid strep test or throat swab culture is performed. Both tests involve gently swabbing the back of the throat close to the tonsils with a cotton swab. A lab test can detect a bacterial infection. A viral infection will not show on the test, but may be assumed if the test for bacteria is negative.

If tests reveal bacteria, treatment will consist of antibiotics to cure the infection. Antibiotics may be given as a single shot or taken 10 days by mouth. Although symptoms will likely improve within two or three days after starting the antibiotic, it's important to take all of the medication to make sure the bacteria are gone. Some people need to take a second course of antibiotics to cure the infection.

If the tonsillitis is caused by a virus, antibiotics will not work and your body will fight off the infection on its own. In the meantime, the following methods can relieve the symptoms, regardless of the cause. They include:

- Get enough rest
- Drink warm or very cold fluids to ease throat pain
- Eat smooth foods, such as flavored gelatins, ice cream, or applesauce
- Use a cool-mist vaporizer or humidifier in your room
- Gargle with warm salt water
- Suck on lozenges containing benzocaine or other anesthetics

- Take over-the-counter pain relievers such as acetaminophen or ibuprofen.

When Tonsillectomy is Needed

If tonsillitis is recurrent or persistent, or if enlarged tonsils cause upper airway obstruction or difficulty eating, surgical removal of the tonsils, called tonsillectomy, may be necessary. Most tonsillectomies involve using a conventional scalpel to remove the tonsils; however there are many alternatives to this traditional method. Increasingly doctors are using techniques such as lasers, radio waves, ultrasonic energy, or electrocautery to cut, burn, or evaporate away enlarged tonsils.

As with all surgeries, each of these has benefits and drawbacks. When considering the procedure, it's important to discuss your options with the surgeon to select the most appropriate one for your child.

The major advantage of removing a child's tonsils is that the operation is much less painful for children than it is for full grown adults. If it becomes necessary to remove the tonsils during adulthood, the convalescence period is about two weeks of severe pain, especially upon swallowing.

What to Expect After Surgery

Tonsillectomy is an outpatient procedure performed under general anesthesia and typically lasting between 30 and 45 minutes. It is most commonly performed in children.

Most children go home about four hours after surgery and require a week to 10 days to recover. Almost all children will have throat pain, ranging from mild to severe, after surgery. Some may experience pain in the ears, jaw, and neck. Medication to ease the pain may be prescribed or recommended.

During the recovery period, it's important for patient to get enough rest. It is also important to make sure patient gets plenty of fluids; however, milk products should be avoided for the first 24 hours after surgery. Although throat pain may make patient reluctant to eat, the sooner a patient eats, the sooner he or she will recover.

For several days after surgery, patients may experience a low-grade fever and small specks of blood from the nose or saliva. If the fever is greater than

102 degrees or if bright red blood is found, a doctor should be called right away. Prompt medical attention may be necessary.

Peritonsillar Abscess

A peritonsillar abscess forms in the tissues of the throat next to one of the tonsils. An abscess is a collection of pus that forms near an area of infected skin or other soft tissue.

The abscess can cause pain, swelling, and, if severe, blockage of the throat. If the throat is blocked, swallowing, speaking, and even breathing can become difficult.

When an infection of the tonsils (known as tonsillitis) spreads and causes infection in the soft tissues, a peritonsillar abscess may result.

Peritonsillar abscess is relatively common in adults but rare in infants and young children.

Etiology

A peritonsillar abscess is most often a complication of tonsillitis. The bacteria involved are similar to those that cause strep throat.

Streptococcal bacteria most commonly cause an infection in the soft tissue around the tonsils (usually just on one side). The tissue is then invaded by anaerobes (bacteria that can live without oxygen), which enter through nearby glands.

- Dental infection (such as the gum infections periodontitis and gingivitis) may be a risk factor. Other risk factors include:
  o Chronic tonsillitis
  o Infectious mononucleosis
  o Smoking
  o Chronic lymphocytic leukemia (CLL)
  o Stones or calcium deposits in the tonsils (tonsilloliths)

Diagnosis and Tests

The first symptom of a peritonsillar abscess is usually a sore throat. A period without fever or other symptoms may follow as the abscess develops. It is not unusual for a delay of 2-5 days between the start of symptoms and abscess formation.

- The mouth and throat may show a swollen area of inflammation -- typically on one side.
- The uvula (the small finger of tissue that hangs down in the middle of the throat) may be shoved away from the swollen side of the mouth.
- Lymph glands in the neck may be enlarged and tender.
- Other signs and symptoms may be observed:
  - Severe sore throat that becomes isolated to one side
  - Painful swallowing
  - Fever and chills
  - Muscle spasm in the muscles of the jaw (trismus) and neck (torticollis)
  - Ear pain on the same side as the abscess
  - A muffled voice, often described as a "hot potato" voice (sounds as if you have a mouthful of hot potato when you talk)
  - Difficulty swallowing saliva

A peritonsillar abscess is usually diagnosed based on history and physical examination. A peritonsillar abscess is easy to diagnose when it is large enough to see. The doctor will look into patient mouth using a light and, possibly, a tongue depressor. Swelling and redness on one side of the throat near the tonsil suggests an abscess. The doctor may also gently push on the area with a gloved finger to see if there is pus from infection inside.

- Lab tests and x-rays are not used often. Sometimes an x-ray or an ultrasound will be performed, typically to make sure other upper airway illnesses are not present. These conditions may include the following:
  - Epiglottitis, an inflammation of the epiglottis (the flap of tissue that prevents food from entering the trachea)
  - Retropharyngeal abscess, a pocket of pus that forms beneath the soft tissue in the back of the throat (like a peritonsillar abscess but in a different location)

o   Peritonsillar cellulitis, an infection of the soft tissue itself (a peritonsillar abscess forms beneath the surface of the tissue)
- The doctor may test patient for mononucleosis, a virus. Some experts suggest that mono is associated with up to 20% of peritonsillar abscesses.

The doctor also may send some of the pus from the abscess to the lab so the exact bacteria can be identified. Even so, identifying the bacteria rarely changes treatment

Treatment and Follow-Up for a Peritonsillar Abscess

Discuss any sore throat with fever or other symptoms with doctor by phone or with an office visit to see if the patient has a peritonsillar abscess.

If patient has a sore throat and trouble swallowing, trouble breathing, difficulty speaking, drooling, or any other signs of potential airway obstruction, patient should seek emergency transportation to a hospital's emergency department.

If patient has a peritonsillar abscess, the doctor's primary concern will be patient breathing and ensuring an open airway. If patient life is in danger because patient throat is blocked, the first step may be to insert a needle in the pus pocket and drain away enough fluid so patient can breathe comfortably.

If a patient's life is not in immediate danger, the doctor will make every effort to keep the procedure as painless as possible. Patient will receive a local anesthetic (like at the dentist) injected into the skin over the abscess and, if necessary, pain medicine and sedation through an IV inserted in patient arm. The doctor will use suction to help patient avoid swallowing pus and blood.

- The doctor has several options for treating patient:
   o   Needle aspiration involves slowly putting a needle into the abscess and withdrawing the pus into a syringe.
   o   Incision and drainage involves using a scalpel to make a small cut in the abscess so pus can drain.
   o   Acute tonsillectomy (having a surgeon remove your tonsils) may be needed if, for some reason, patient cannot tolerate a drainage procedure, or if patient have a history of frequent tonsillitis.
- Patient will receive an antibiotic. The first dose may be given through an IV. Penicillin is the best drug for this type of infection, but if

patient is allergic, another antibiotic may be used (other choices may be erythromycin or clindamycin).

- If patient is healthy and the abscess drains well, the patient can go home. If the patient is very ill, cannot swallow, or has complicating medical problems (such as diabetes), the patient may be admitted to the hospital. Young children, who often need general anesthesia for drainage, frequently require a hospital stay for observation.

Arrange follow-up with the operating doctor or an ear-nose-throat specialist (otolaryngologist) after treatment for a peritonsillar abscess. Also:

- If the abscess starts to return, patient may need a different antibiotic or further drainage.
- If patient develop excessive bleeding or have trouble breathing or swallowing, seek medical attention immediately.

Prevention of a Peritonsillar Abscess

There is no reliable method for preventing a peritonsillar abscess other than reducing risks: Do not smoke, maintain good dental hygiene, and promptly treat oral infections.

- If a patient develops peritonsillar cellulitis, the patient may possibly prevent a peritonsillar abscess by taking an antibiotic. However, the patient should be closely monitored for abscess formation and may even be hospitalized.
- If a patient is likely to form an abscess (for example, if the patient have tonsillitis frequently), he or she should talk with a doctor about whether the patient should have a tonsillectomy.
- As with any prescription, the patient must finish the full course of the antibiotic even if the patient feels better after a few days.

Outlook for a Peritonsillar Abscess

People with an uncomplicated, well-treated peritonsillar abscess usually recover fully. If a patient does not have chronic tonsillitis, the chance of the abscess returning is only 10%, and removing the tonsils is usually not necessary.

Most complications occur in people with diabetes, in people whose immune systems are weakened (such as those with AIDS, transplant recipients on immune-suppressing drugs, or cancer patients), or in those who fail to recognize the seriousness of the illness and do not seek medical attention.

- Major complications of a peritonsillar abscess include:
  o Airway blockage
  o Bleeding from erosion of the abscess into a major blood vessel
  o Dehydration from difficulty swallowing
  o Infection in the tissues beneath the breastbone
  o Pneumonia
  o Meningitis
  o Sepsis (bacteria in the bloodstream)

- Acute mononucleosis: Usually caused by the Epstein-Barr virus, "mono" causes severe swelling in the tonsils, fever, sore throat, rash, and fatigue.
- Strep throat: *Streptococcus*, a bacterium, infects the tonsils and throat. Fever and neck pain often accompany the sore throat.
- Enlarged (hypertrophic) tonsils: Large tonsils reduce the size of the airway, making snoring or sleep apnea more likely.
- Tonsilloliths (tonsil stones): Tonsil stones, or tonsilloliths, are formed when this trapped debris hardens, or calcifies.

Tonsillar Hypertrophy

Tonsillar hypertrophy is the enlargement of the tonsils, but without a history of inflammation and obstructive tonsillar hypertrophy is currently the most common reason for tonsillectomy. These patients usually present with varying degrees of disturbed sleep which may include symptoms of loud snoring, irregular breathing, nocturnal choking and coughing, frequent awakenings, sleep apnea, dysphagia (pain on eating) and/or daytime hypersomnolence. These may lead to behavioral/mood changes in patients and facilitate the need for a polysomnography (sleep evaluation) in order to determine the degree to which these symptoms are disrupting their sleep.

Tonsiloliths (Tonsil Stones)

People with chronic sinusitis and post nasal drip may develop tonsiloliths, which are tiny, white, foul smelling stones which lodge in the tonsilar crypts. Sometimes a tonsolith can be pried out of the surface of the tonsil with a pencil or other small pointed instrument leaving what appears to be a little "hole" but is, in actuality, the tonsilar crypt in which it originally formed. Tonsiloliths sometimes give the feeling of something lodged in the throat. They can also contribute to bad breath. Some people have chronic problems with tonsiloliths. The only sure treatment for chronic tonsiloliths is removal of the tonsils. The operation is performed by an ear, nose and throat specialist (ENT) and is fairly simple and safe. As noted above, in adults the operation causes a very serious sore throat for two weeks post-op. Short of removing the tonsils, the bad breath can be treated with mouth rinses, and the condition itself may be lessened by gargling with Peridex® mouth wash which is available by prescription from your dentist or physician, and possibly by the use of decongestants to lessen the post nasal drip which is part of the cause of tonsiloliths.

In: Tonsillar Disorders   ISBN: 978-1-61209-275-1
Editor: Anne C. Hallberg   ©2011 Nova Science Publishers, Inc.

Chapter V

Post-Tonsillectomy Hemorrhage

Olaf Zagólski

Affiliation: St. John Grande's Hospital, Kraków, Poland

Abstract

The most serious complication of tonsillectomy is bleeding. Primary post-tonsillectomy hemorrhage (PTH) occurs during the first 24 hours following the procedure, usually as a consequence of inadequate ligation of the feeding arteries. Secondary PTH occurs most frequently between the 5-8 postoperative days. Incidence of such episodes counts in several percent being an important clinical problem due to the number of tonsillectomies being very frequently performed ENT procedures. PTH occurs significantly more frequently in adults (age equal to or above 15 years) than in children. In children, the risk is higher in boys and in individuals with frequent infections of the tonsils. In adult patients, peritonsillar abscess as indication for surgery increases the risk of PTH. Bleeding occurs more frequently after "hot" than "cold" technique and the use of coblation significantly increases the occurrence of PTH. Cryptic tonsillitis and actinomyces infection diagnosed on histopathological examination of tonsillar tissue were found to correlate with PTH, whereas patient's gender and season of surgery were not. Performing tonsillectomy in warmer weather when water vapor pressure is higher may reduce secondary hemorrhage rate. Incidence of secondary PTH does not depend on post-operative infection. Post-tonsillectomy hemorrhage rate significantly correlates with personal history of proneness to bruise formation and proneness to prolonged bleeding after minor injuries. In rare cases, the intensity of PTH may become life-threatening and requires major surgical means and intensive care.

Introduction

The most serious complication of tonsillectomy is bleeding [1-3]. Primary post-tonsillectomy hemorrhage (PTH) occurs during the first 24 hours following the procedure, usually as a consequence of inadequate ligation of the feeding arteries [4, 5]. It has been observed that the longer ambulatory tonsillectomy lasts, the greater risk of primary PTH [6]. Secondary PTH occurs most frequently between the 5-8 postoperative days [2, 4, 5, 7-9]. Debridement of the fibrin layers is generally considered the cause [5]. Incidence of such episodes counts in several percent being an important clinical problem due to the number of tonsillectomies, which are very frequently performed ENT procedures [2, 3, 8, 10, 11].

Incidence and Risk Factors of Post-Tonsillectomy Hemorrhage

PTH has been a subject of numerous clinical studies aiming to establish its causes and ways of avoiding it. Criteria for recognizing serious bleeding are either 1) repeat anesthesia and surgery because of hemorrhage (including return to theater from the recovery room), or 2) readmission to hospital because of bleeding, or 3) blood transfusion to replace blood loss [11]. Minor hemorrhages subside spontaneously. Main measures of PTH are the incidence, volume, and time course of postoperative hemorrhage [12]. In many countries, including the United States, tonsillectomy has been performed in healthy patients as ambulatory procedure [11]. In some European countries, including Germany, tonsillectomy-patients are kept as inpatients until the fifth to seventh day after surgery to care for pain-management, food-intake and possible hemorrhage [5]. Rates of PTH vary between different institutions. In the Department of Otolaryngology, Head and Neck Surgery, Karolinska University Hospital, 212 (7.5%) patients were readmitted due to PTH, of which 98 (3.4%) presented with ongoing hemorrhage. The rates of primary and secondary bleeding were 1.9 and 5.5%, respectively. The PTH occurred in

0-19 days post-operatively, in a typical twin peak mode around the day of surgery and then days 4-7. No case of serious PTH was noted. Multiple bleedings (2-3 times) occurred in 19 patients. Only a minority (31%) of the single PTH patients required active treatment, surgery in the theatre (35 patients) or diathermy under local anesthesia in the emergency room (24 patients). However, almost all received systemic haemostatic treatment. Three patients required blood transfusion due to repeated PTH. Of the 114 patients that did not present with an active PTH, only 1 returned to the operating theatre due to later bleeding. Almost half (43%) of the patients with multiple episodes of PTH had also experienced primary bleedings. The authors conclude that a primary PTH seems to indicate a risk of further episodes of bleedings, and should necessitate extra post-operative observation. Patients with a history of a single self-limiting PTH showed low risk of developing a hemorrhage requiring return to the theatre [11, 13]. Hemorrhage risk after quinsy tonsillectomy was the subject of research conducted at Department of Oto-Rhino-Laryngology-Head and Neck Surgery, Geneva University Hospital, Geneva, Switzerland [14]. Bleeding occurred in 27 patients (13%). Ipsilateral hemorrhage was observed in 8 patients (4%) and contralateral hemorrhage in 19 patients (9%). The higher incidence of PTH in the side contralateral to the abscess was found to be statistically significant ($P = 0.02$). Male gender ($P = 0.042$), smoking ($P = 0.009$), and aspirin intake ($P = 0.008$) were statistically significant factors associated with an increased PTH risk in this groups of patients [14]. The risk of bleeding following abscess tonsillectomy seemed higher than reported in elective tonsillectomy [14, 15]. This high incidence was mainly due to patients with prior aspirin intake or to bleeding in the side contralateral to the abscess. The authors suggest that postoperative bleeding could be reduced by performing a unilateral acute abscess tonsillectomy in selected patients [14]. Bleeding occurs more frequently after "hot" than "cold" technique and the use of coblation significantly increases the occurrence of PTH [4, 12, 15-17]. Coblation procedures performed by non-experienced surgeons are substantially more frequently complicated with hemorrhage [15]. Gold laser tonsillectomy has hemorrhage rate similar to cold steel dissection and lower than coblation tonsillectomy [18]. The efficacy and safety of radiofrequency and monopolar electrocautery tonsillectomy, regarding tonsillectomy morbidity, including PTH, was examined at Department of Otorhinolaryngology and Head and Neck Surgery, Haseki Research and Training Hospital, Istanbul, Turkey. The mean +/- standard deviation of the operation duration required for the radiofrequency method was significantly longer than that for monopolar electrocautery: 8.1 +/- 1.6 minutes vs 7.3 +/-

1.5 minutes, respectively (p = 0.034). PTH was observed in only three patients (13.6 per cent). Inter-group analysis showed no significant differences in post-operative pain scores for the radiofrequency vs monopolar electrocautery methods (3.7 +/- 1.6 vs 3.3 +/- 1.4, respectively; p < 0.126). Inter-group analysis showed that tonsillar fossa wound healing scores evaluated on the fifth, 10th and 14th post-operative days were significantly higher in the radiofrequency group compared with the monopolar electrocautery group (p < 0.001). The authors observed that monopolar electrocautery tonsillectomy was superior to radiofrequency tonsillectomy in terms of post-operative tonsillar fossa wound healing; however, both techniques were comparable in terms of post-operative pain [19]. The incidence and pattern of bleeding after tonsillectomy performed by either cold dissection or diathermy was the subject of a clinical trial at the Department of Otolaryngology, The University of Melbourne, Royal Victorian Eye and Ear Hospital, Victoria, Australia [12]. The number of bilateral tonsillectomies with removal by cold-blunt dissection was 3,087. In this group, there were 57 (1.85%) bleeds. The number of bilateral tonsillectomies with removal by diathermy dissection was 1,557. In this group, there were 37 (2.38%) bleeds. If cold dissection is taken as the "control" and diathermy tonsillectomy as the "treatment" group, the relative risk of bleeding after diathermy tonsillectomy is 1.30 (95% confidence interval 0.88-1.93). The pattern of bleeding after each technique differed significantly over time, with more reactionary bleeds in the dissection group and more bleeds between 4 to 7 postoperative days after diathermy. When bleeding occurred, it was in excess of 500 mL in 16% of dissection cases and 43% of diathermy tonsillectomies. The difference in the risk of bleeding after each technique did not reach statistical significance, but the temporal pattern of hemorrhage differed, and more bleeds exceeding 500 mL were seen in the diathermy group [12]. The study conducted at Department of Otolaryngology, Ninewells Hospital and Medical School, Dundee, UK aimed to determine whether bipolar dissection tonsillectomy is associated with a higher post-operative hemorrhage rate than cold dissection tonsillectomy [17]. The hemorrhage rates for procedures conducted by senior house officers, specialist registrars and consultants were 11.4 per cent, 10.3 per cent and 5.0 per cent, respectively. Two patients required surgical intervention, both from the bipolar dissection group. No patients required blood transfusion. A history of quinsy was not associated with an increased hemorrhage rate [17]. The difference in hemorrhage rates between groups and surgeon grades did not reach statistical significance. Nonetheless the trend towards a greater incidence of hemorrhage in the bipolar group and in procedures conducted by more junior surgeons during the trial raised concerns and disallowed the use of bipolar dissection in tonsillectomies performed by junior staff members [17]. A survey conveyed at Surgery and Paediatrics, University of Newcastle, Newcastle, NSW, Australia involved one thousand one hundred thirty-three consecutive cases of tonsillectomy. The primary post-tonsillectomy hemorrhage rate was 0.2% for blunt dissection plus diathermy hemostasis and 0.3% for monopolar diathermy dissection plus hemostasis. Monopolar diathermy had a lower rate of secondary postoperative hemorrhage, requiring readmission (4.2% compared with 5.4% for blunt dissection plus diathermy hemostasis) and a lower rate for readmission for observation alone (2.1% compared with 4.2%) but had a higher risk of returning to surgery (1.6% compared with 1.04%) and a higher risk of blood transfusion (0.49% compared with 0.2%). These differences, however, did not reach statistical significance (Yates chi(2)), and neither did the relative risk between the two techniques. Two-way analysis of variance among secondary post-tonsillectomy hemorrhage complications by technique and by age groups shows a highly statistically significant difference by age group (analysis of variance, 3 df, $F = 9.509$, $P < 0.001$), much more so than technique [16]. PTH occurs significantly more frequently in adults (age equal to or above 15 years) than in children [15, 20]. In children, the risk of PTH is higher in boys [20]. Patients who undergo tonsillectomy for chronic tonsillar infection have an increased incidence of postoperative bleeding [3]. Incidence of secondary PTH does not depend on post-operative infection [21]. Correspondingly, the routine use of antibiotics should be questioned for secondary tonsillectomy hemorrhage [21]. Cryptic tonsillitis and actinomyces infection diagnosed on histopathological examination of tonsillar tissue were found to correlate with PTH, whereas patient's gender and season of surgery were not [1]. Performing tonsillectomy in warmer weather when water vapor pressure is higher may reduce secondary hemorrhage rate [22]. Synchronous nasal surgery does not increase the rate of PTH [23]. Blood type-O is associated with decreased expression of von Willebrand factor. Type-O patients suffer fewer thrombotic problems and may be more prone to hemorrhages. Blood group O is disproportionately represented in secondary post-tonsillectomy hemorrhage patients and might be responsible for a count of the cases [24]. The occurrence of post-tonsillectomy hemorrhage does not increase in patients with significant family history of coagulation disorders. Personal history of recurrent epistaxis, bruises after minor trauma and prolonged bleeding after minor injury are significant for post-tonsillectomy hemorrhage [25]. Seasonal variation in post-tonsillectomy hemorrhages was not found [26].

Life-Threatening Hemorrhages

In rare cases, the intensity of PTH may become life-threatening and requires major surgical means and intensive care [27]. Cases occurring during the clinical career of the authors at Department of Otorhinolaryngology, St. Anna Krankenhaus, Duisburg, Germany were collected and added by own expert reports to lawsuits and professional boards in cases who had undergone tonsillectomy elsewhere. PTH resulting in hemorrhagic shock requiring resuscitation, ligature of greater arteries in the neck, tracheotomy, packing of the pharynx, embolization, and/or blood transfusions were labeled as life threatening. Seventy-nine patients had experienced life-threatening PTH between 1980 and 2006, comprising 36 children and 39 adults (age not stated for 4 patients). There were 42 female and 34 male patients (gender not stated for 3 patients). Only nine patients experienced primary bleeding, secondary PTH clearly prevailed (n = 70; 89.6%) in this patient population. Single episodes of life-threatening PTH were reported for 11 cases including two patients with and nine without remaining neurological sequels. Three of the 11 patients were children (age not stated for 2 patients). Repeated episodes of life-threatening PTH occurred in 68 patients (32 children) including eight with remaining sequels. Life-threatening PTH is an apparently rare, most commonly unpredictable state of emergency requiring a clear management protocol. However, repeated episodes of bleeding classified most clinical courses and should alert the medical staff. Although the bleeding rate after tonsillectomy in children is generally acknowledged to be very low, the rate of life-threatening PTH is apparently higher than in adults. Gender seems not to be a risk factor. Secondary PTH can no longer be assessed to be less dangerous than primary PTH [27].

Coagulation and Post-Tonsillectomy Hemorrhage

Preoperative evaluation of coagulation is performed in order to predict possibility of hemorrhage during and after surgery [4]. Among the coagulation tests, activated partial thromboplastin time (APTT), prothrombin time and platelet count have been routinely assessed [7, 10]. APTT reflects activity of plasma clotting factors VIII, IX, XI and XII that constitute endogenous system of prothrombin activation. Value of APTT depends on the activity of factors participating in thrombin generation and transformation of fibrinogen into fibrin. Normal values are between 26 and 36 s. APTT is prolonged in case of factors V, VIII, IX, X and XI, prothrombin, fibrinogen, and vitamin K deficiency [4, 10]. Prothrombin time value represents exogenous coagulation system function and depends on blood concentration of the factors II, V, VII, X and fibrinogen. Prothrombin time is commonly expressed as international normalized ratio – INR and its normal values are between 0.9 and 1.3 [4, 10]. Several recent studies concluded that performing routine coagulation tests does not have predictive value for the occurrence of PTH, at least in children [2, 7, 28]. Detailed family history and preoperative history of coagulation disorders proved sensitive in disclosing hidden coagulopathies in young patients in whom tonsillectomy is indicated [2, 4]. Detailed medical history of coagulation disorders has been found to correlate with incidence of PTH in children [2, 4]. Therefore universal preoperative hematological screening does not seem to be cost-effective [4, 25]. If the family history and also both the preoperative history and detailed physical examination are suspicious, e.g. recurrent mild nasal bleeding, hidden coagulopathy needs to be ruled out [4, 25]. Non-steriodal anti-inflammatory drugs (Ibuprofen, Diclofenac) are not a contraindication to tonsillectomy and should be used in the control of postoperative pain if it is indicated in the patient [29, 30].

Treatment of Post-Tonsillectomy Hemorrhage

Many minor PTHs resolve spontaneously. In persistent PTH, reintubation of the patient is necessary which might be challenging due to presence of blood in the upper respiratory tract and worsening condition of the patient [13]. Reintubation is inevitable in all patients with the hemorrhage site difficult to localize. If the bleeding site is evident, electrocautery under local anesthesia can be performed and is usually sufficient [5]. If bleeding persists, tonsillar beds must be stitched on a swab.

Conclusion

A primary PTH seems to indicate elevated risk of further episodes of bleedings. The risk of bleeding following abscess tonsillectomy seemed higher than reported in elective tonsillectomy. Bleeding occurs more frequently after "hot" than "cold" technique and the use of coblation significantly increases the occurrence of PTH. Experience of the surgeon is of crucial importance in avoiding PTH. Patients who undergo tonsillectomy for chronic tonsillar infection have an increased incidence of postoperative bleeding. Incidence of secondary PTH does not depend on post-operative infection. Blood type-O is associated with increased PTH rate. Performing routine coagulation tests does not have predictive value for the occurrence of PTH, at least in children. History of recurrent epistaxis, bruises after minor trauma and prolonged bleeding after minor injury are significant for PTH. Non-steriodal anti-inflammatory drugs are not a contraindication to tonsillectomy and should be used in the control of postoperative pain if it is indicated in the patient

References

[1]   Schrock, A; Send, T; Heukamp, L; Gerstner, AO; Bootz, F; Jakob, M. The role of histology and other risk factors for post-tonsillectomy haemorrhage. *Eur Arch Otorhinolaryngol.* 2009, 226, 1983-7.

[2]   Stuck, BA; Genzwürker, HV. Tonsillectomy in children : Preoperative evaluation of risk factors. *Anaesthesist* 2008, 57, 499-504.

[3]   Hoddeson, EK; Gourin, CG. Adult tonsillectomy: current indications and outcomes. *Otolaryngol Head Neck Surg.* 2009, 140, 19-22.

[4]   Gerlinger, I; Török, L; Nagy, A; Patzkó, A; Losonczy, H; Pytel, J. Frequency of coagulopathies in cases with post-tonsillectomy bleeding. *Orv Hetil.* 2008, 149, 441-6.

[5]   Deitmer, T; Neuwirth, C.105 Cases of Post-Tonsillectomy Hemorrhage Revisited. *Laryngorhinootologie*, in press.

[6]   Ahmad, R; Abdullah, K; Amin, Z; Rahman, JA. Predicting safe tonsillectomy for ambulatory surgery. *Auris Nasus Larynx* 2010, 37, 185-9.

[7]   Eisert, S; Hovermann, M; Bier, H; Göbel, U. Preoperative screening for coagulation disorders in children undergoing adenoidectomy (AT) and

tonsillectomy (TE): does it prevent bleeding complications? Klin Padiatr. 2006, 218, 334-9.

[8] Johnson, LB; Elluru, RC; Myer, CM 3rd. Complications of adenotonsillectomy. *Laryngoscope* 2002, ll2, 35-6.

[9] Smith, SL; Pereira, KD. Tonsillectomy in children: indications, diagnosis and complications. *ORL J Otorhinolaryngol Relat Spec.* 2007, 69, 336-9.

[10] Scheckenbach, K; Bier, H; Hoffmann, TK; Windfuhr, JP; Bas, M; Laws, HJ; Plettenberg, C; Wagenmann, M. Risk of hemorrhage after adenoidectomy and tonsillectomy: value of the preoperative determination of partial thromboplastin time, prothrombin time and platelet count. HNO. 2008, 56, 312-20.

[11] Attner, P; Haraldsson, PO; Hemlin, C; Hessén Soderman, AC. A 4-year consecutive study of post-tonsillectomy haemorrhage. *ORL J Otorhinolaryngol Relat Spec.* 2009, 71, 273-8.

[12] O'Leary, S; Vorrath, J. Postoperative bleeding after diathermy and dissection tonsillectomy. *Laryngoscope* 2005, 115, 591-4.

[13] Brar, MS. Airway management in a bleeding adult following tonsillectomy: a case report. *AANA J.* 2009, 77, 428-30.

[14] Giger, R; Landis, BN; Dulguerov, P. Hemorrhage risk after quinsy tonsillectomy. *Otolaryngol Head Neck Surg.* 2005, 133, 729-34.

[15] Heidemann, CH; Wallén, M; Aakesson, M; Skov, P; Kjeldsen, AD; Godballe, C. Post-tonsillectomy hemorrhage: assessment of risk factors with special attention to introduction of coblation technique. *Eur Arch Otorhinolaryngol.* 2009, 266, 1011-5.

[16] Walker, P; Gillies, D. Post-tonsillectomy hemorrhage rates: Are they technique-dependent? *Otolaryngol Head Neck Surg.* 2007, 136, 27-31.

[17] Haddow, K; Montague, ML; Hussain, SS. Post-tonsillectomy haemorrhage: a prospective, randomized, controlled clinical trial of cold dissection versus bipolar diathermy dissection. *J Laryngol Otol.* 2006, 120, 450-4.

[18] Giles, JE; Worley, NK; Telusca, N.Gold laser tonsillectomy--a safe new method. *Int J Pediatr Otorhinolaryngol.* 2009, 73, 1274-7.

[19] Aksoy, F; Ozturan, O; Veyseller, B; Yildirim, YS; Demirhan, H.Comparison of radiofrequency and monopolar electrocautery tonsillectomy. *J Laryngol Otol.* 2010, 124, 180-4.

[20] Windfuhr, JP; Chen YS. Incidence of post-tonsillectomy hemorrhage in children and adults: a study of 4,848 patients. *Ear Nose Throat J.* 2002, 81, 626-8.

[21] Ahsan, F; Rashid, H; Eng, C; Bennett, DM; Ah-See, KW. Is secondary haemorrhage after tonsillectomy in adults an infective condition? Objective measures of infection in a prospective cohort. *Clin Otolaryngol.* 2007, 32, 24-7.

[22] Lee, MS; Montague, ML; Hussain, SS. The influence of weather on the frequency of secondary post-tonsillectomy haemorrhage. *J Laryngol Otol.* 2005, 119, 894-8.

[23] Adams, MT; Wilhelm, MJ; Demars, SM; Harsha, WJ. Effects of synchronous nasal surgery on posttonsillectomy hemorrhage. *Arch Otolaryngol Head Neck Surg.* 2009, 135, 936-9.

[24] Leonard, DS; Fenton, JE; Hone, S. ABO blood type as a risk factor for secondary post-tonsillectomy haemorrhage. *Int J Pediatr Otorhinolaryngol.*, in press.

[25] Zagólski, O. Post-tonsillectomy haemorrhage-Do coagulation tests and coagulopathy history have predictive value? *Acta Otorrinolaringol Esp.*, in press

[26] Kvaerner, KJ. Benchmarking surgery: secondary post-tonsillectomy hemorrhage 1999-2005. *Acta Otolaryngol.* 2009, 129, 195-8.

[27] Windfuhr, JP; Schloendorff, G; Baburi, D; Kremer, B. Life-threatening posttonsillectomy hemorrhage. *Laryngoscope* 2008, 118, 1389-94.

[28] Eberl, W; Wendt, I; Schroeder, HG. Preoperative coagulation screening prior to adenoidectomy and tonsillectomy. *Klin Padiatr.* 2005, 217, 20-4.

[29] Jeyakumar, A; Brickman, TM; Williamson, ME; Hirose, K; Krakovitz, P; Whittemore, K; Discolo, C. Nonsteroidal anti-inflammatory drugs and postoperative bleeding following adenotonsillectomy in pediatric patients. *Arch Otolaryngol Head Neck Surg.* 2008, 134, 24-7.

[30] Heaney, M; Looney, Y; McKinstry, C; O'Hare, B.Sequential clot strength analyses following diclofenac in pediatric adenotonsillectomy. *Paediatr Anaesth.* 2007, 17, 1078-82.

In: Tonsillar Disorders
Editor: Anne C. Hallberg

ISBN: 978-1-61209-275-1
©2011 Nova Science Publishers, Inc.

Chapter VI

Distribution of Tumor Necrosis Factor Producing Cells in Chronic Tonsillitis[*]

Milan Stankovic[†1], Miroljub Todorovic[2],
Verica Avramovic[3], Misa Vlahovic[4]
and Dragan Mihailovic[5]

[1]ORL Clinic Nis, University Clinical Center Nis, Serbia,
[2]ORL Clinic Cetinje, University Clinical Center Podgorica, Montenegro,
[3]Institute for Histology, Medical Faculty Nis, Serbia,
[4]Clinic for Nephrology, University Clinical Center Nis, Serbia,
[5]Institute for Pathology, University Clinical Center Nis, Serbia

---

[*] A version of this chapter was also published in *Handbook of Pharyngeal Diseases: Etiology, Diagnosis and Treatment,* edited by Aaron P. Nazario and Julien K. Vermeulen, published by Nova Science Publishers, Inc. It was submitted for appropriate modifications in an effort to encourage wider dissemination of research.

[†] Correspondence: Milan Stankovic, ORL Clinic Nis, Bul. Z. Djindjica 48, 18 000 Nis, Serbia, Tel. +381 18 520 595, E-mail: milan.orl@bankerinter.net

Abstract

Objective: is to determine and quantify the production of TNF-α in chronic tonsillitis.

Material and methods: The study comprised of 23 patients with chronic tonsillitis, divided in two groups: 10 patients with tonsillar hypertrophy (TH) with average age 9.0 ± 2.7 years, and 13 patients with recurrent tonsillitis (RT) aged 23.1 ± 5.2 years.

Highly sensitive labeled streptavidin-biotin horse reddish peroxidase immunohistochemical method (LSAB+/HRP) was used for detection of TNF-α producing cells. Quantification of TNF-α was made for crypt epithelium, germinative centers, roundness of follicles, interfollicular areas and subepithelial area. Quantification of lymph follicles and germinative centers included: areal (mm2), median optical density (au), circumference (mm), Ferret diameter (mm), and integrated optical density (IOD).

Results: Distribution of TNF-α producing cells is similar for TH and RT. They are mainly found in subepithelial areas, interfollicular regions, and germinative centers of lymph follicles, and rarely in crypt epithelium. Numerical density of TNF-α producing cells is significantly higher in RT, compared to TH.

Conclusion: Quantification of TNF-α producing cells confirm domination of cellular Th1 immune response both in TH and RT.

Keywords: tonsillar hypertrophy, recurrent tonsillitis, tumor necrosis factor, morphometry

Introduction

Palatine tonsil is involved in active production of cytokines. This soluble protein have a key role in immunity and inflammatory reactions. According to the subtype of cytokine producing T lymphocyte, and the role in immune reactions, they are divided on Th1 and Th2, as well as on proinflammatory and anti-inflammatory cytokines. Tumor necrosis factor (TNF-α) is a cytokine that is important for immune response and allergic reactions [1]. TNF-α is a mediator of local inflammatory response causing cascade reaction of cytokines, increased vascular permeability, and enables accumulation of macrophages and neutophyles [2].

It was confirmed that palatine tonsils produce both Th1 (interleukin-2, interferon-γ, TNF-α), and Th2 (interleukin 4, 5, 6, and 13) with predomination Th1 cytokines [3-8]. During infections Th1 cytokines are the first to be produced, with later formation of Th2 type. [9-10] Production of cytokines in tonsillar mononuclear cells is amplified after stimulation with mitogen, or antigen [6, 9, 10]. Cytokines from palatine tonsils are regulators and modulators of immune response on pathogenic agents, especially during acute phase, and in repeated infections. [3]

The aim of the present study is to determine and quantify the presence of TNF-α producing cells, as a representative of Th1 cytokines, in chronic tonsillitis.

Materials and Methods

The study comprised of 23 patients with chronic tonsillitis, divided in two groups: 10 patients with tonsillar hypertrophy (TH) with average age 9.0 ± 2.7 years, and 13 patients with recurrent tonsillitis (RT) aged 23.1 ± 5.2 years [11].

Indications for tonsillectomy were based on anamnesis, clinical presentation and laboratory tests. During surgical treatment the patients were without acute infection or antibiotic treatment. Removed palatine tonsils were rinsed in physiological saline, and fixed for 24 hours in buffered for-maldehyde.

Highly sensitive labeled streptavidin-biotin horse reddish peroxidase immunohistochemical method (LSAB+/HRP) was used for detection of TNF-α producing cells. Monoclonal anti-human antibodies, and 3,3`-diamino-bensidine as chromogen were applied. Tonsillar slices 4 μm thick were mounted on adherent plates (Super Frost Plus, Menzel-Glaser, Deutschland), dried for one hour at 56^0C. Primary antisera were diluted (DAKO Antibody diluent, S0809, Denmark). Tissue samples were deparafined, and rehydrated under pressure for 2 minutes in 0.01M citrate buffer, pH 6 (Target Retrival Solution, S 1700, DAKO). After unmasking the antigens, endogen paroxydase was blocked using 3% aqueous H_2O_2 for 10 minutes at room temperature. Incubation with primary antigen (60 minutes), than incubation with biotinized anti-goat immunoglobulin (30 minutes), and incubation with streptavidine conjugate (30 minutes) were than performed. For visualization of antigen-antibody complex we used 3-amino-9-etilcarbasol (DAKO AEC+ Substrate /

Chromogen System, 01475) for 10 minutes. Meyer hematoxylin (Merck, Deutschland) served for nuclear dying. Control of quality and specificity of process was tested using positive and negative control (UK National External Quality Assessment for Immunocytochemistry) [12].

Quantification of TNF-α was made on the same tissue samples, separately for crypt epithelium, germinative centers, roundness of follicles, interfollicular areas and subepithelial area. Digital pictures 1280x960 pixels using microscope NU-2 (Carl Zeiss, Jena), with objective x25 (NA=0.50), and web camera MSI 370i with test area 0.02 mm^2 were used. Numerical areal density (N_A) was calculated according to formula: $N_A=N/A_t$ (N- number of TNF-α cells, A_t- test area). Numerical volume (N_V) represented: $N_V=N_A/(t+D-2h)$, (t- thickness of sample, D- diameter of TNF-α cells amounting 13 μm, h- height amounting 2 μm). The number of digital pictures for testing was calculated according to formula: $n=(20s/x^-)^2$, where: s-standard deviation of numerical density, x^-- mean numeric density, and it amounted 240 [13].

Quantification of lymph follicles and germinative centers included: areal (mm^2), median optical density (au), circumference (mm), Feret`s diameter (mm), and integrated optical density (IOD). They were determined using objective x4 (NA=0.1), Image J program of manually edited picture on 70 areas, according to previous formula.

Statistical analyze was performed using SIGMASTAT and ORIGIN programs. Statistical significance was determined with Student`s t test, ANOVA test, and Mann-Whitney Rank sum test.

Results

In tonsillar hypertrophy (TH) TNF-α producing cells were present predominantly in subepithelial areas, on the border between crypt epithelium and subepithelial lymphatic tissue. Intraepithelial localization was rare. On the other side, nearly all germinative centers of enlarged lymph follicles contained TNF-α cells. Interfollicular areas and connective septa had occasional TNF-α cells. Mantle areas were without signs of their presence (Fig. 1-3.).

In recurrent tonsillitis (RT) TNF-α producing cells were mostly found in subepithelial areas as cellular aggregates and bands. They are also present in interfollicular areas towards crypt epithelium, whereas in lymph follicles and intraepithelially they were scant. Germinative centers contain small number of

TNF-α cells. At the border of germinative centers and mantle areas their distribution is linear, forming rings (Fig. 4-6.).

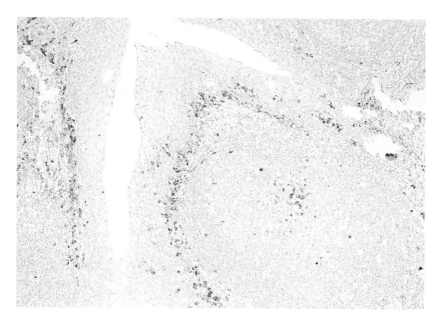

Figure. 1. Tonsillar hypertrophy. TNF-α producing cells are localized subepithelially, group of cells in germinative center, occasional cells are present in crypt epithelium and in interfollicular areas (LSAB/HRP x100).

Figure. 2. Tonsillar hypertrophy. Numerous TNF-α producing cells seen in germinative centers, rare cells are near connective septa (LSAB/HRP x100).

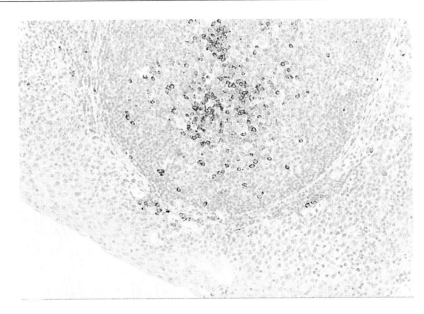

Figure. 3. Tonsillar hypertrophy. TNF-α producing cells mainly in germinative centers, few cells in mantle area (LSAB/HRP x200).

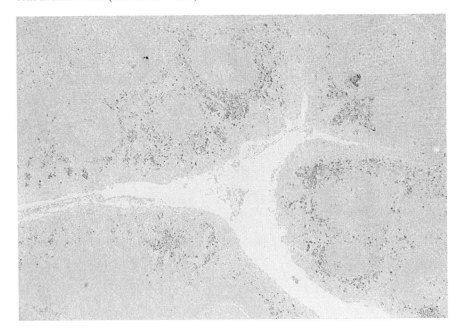

Figure. 4. Recurrent tonsillitis. Visible lymph follicles. TNF-α producing cells are located subepithelially, ratricularly towards crypt epithelium (LSAB/HRP x50).

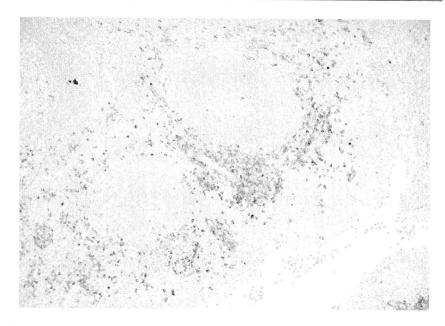

Figure. 5. Recurrent tonsillitis. TNF-α producing cells seen mainly around lymph follicles and subepithelially, rarely in crypt epithelium (LSAB/HRP x100).

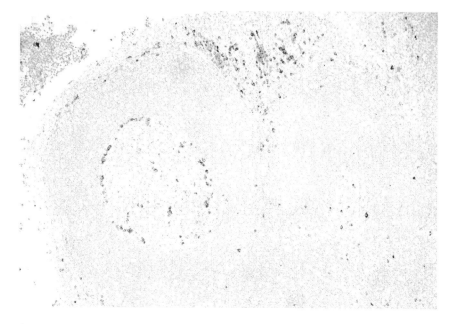

Figure. 6. Recurrent tonsillitis. TNF-α producing cells are visible subepithelially and at the border of germinative centers and mantle areas (LSAB/HRP x100).

Quantification of TNF-α producing cells indicated on statistical significance for numerical areal density (N_A) (ANOVA, Wilks lambda 0.46; Rao R 27.91). Student's t test confirmed highly significant differences of N_A for crypt epithelium and interfollicular areas, as well as significant differences of N_A for subepithelial areas, but not for germinative centers in TH compared to RT (Table 1.). Subepithelial areas and germinative centers were the sites with predominant presence of TNF-α producing cells in both groups of patients (56% for TH and 52% for RT in subepithelial areas; 35% for TH and 25% for RT in germinative centers), with their significantly higher number in interfollicular regions for RT and reduced number in germinative centers.

Table. 1. Numerical areal density (N_A) of TNF-α producing cells (mean ± standard deviation) in tonsillar hypertrophy (TH) and recurrent tonsillitis (RT).

MORPHOLOGICAL AREA	TH	RT	p <
Crypt epithelium	67.3 ± 20.8	117.0 ± 37.5	0.01
Germinative center	1652.7 ± 479.3	1526.1 ± 442.6	0.51
Interfollicular area	436.4 ± 148.4	1298.9 ± 293.8	0.001
Subepithelial area	2661.8 ± 485.9	3121.6 ± 556.9	0.05

Numerical volume density (N_V) of TNF-α producing cells confirmed highly significant differences for interfollicular regions, significant for crypt epithelium and subepithelial regions, but not for germinative centers (Table 2.) Percentual distribution of TNF-α producing cells was adequate to analyze of N_A.

Table. 2. Numerical volume density (N_v) of TNF-α producing cells (mean ± standard deviation) in tonsillar hypertrophy (TH) and recurrent tonsillitis (RT).

MORPHOLOGICAL AREA	TH	RT	p <
Crypt epithelium	4851.8 ± 1358.5	8152.2 ± 2282.6	0.01
Germinative center	119137.5 ± 38124.0	108152.2 ± 34608.7	0.47
Interfollicular area	31603.8 ± 8849.1	70962.7 ± 19869.6	0.001
Subepithelial area	188881.4 ± 26553.2	222981.4 ± 39123.2	0.05

Quantification of size of lymph follicles and their germinative centers resulted in significant differences between TH and RT for all analyzed parameters, except for roundness of follicles. Areal, circumference, diameter, and integrated optical density of lymph follicles were significantly higher in TH compared to RT, while optical density showed inversed values (Table 3.).

Table. 3. Quantification of lymph follicles (mean ± standard deviation) in tonsillar hypertrophy (TH) and recurrent tonsillitis (RT).

PARAMETERS	TH	RT	$p <$
Areal (mm^2)	0.32 ± 0.09	0.20 ± 0.06	0.001
Optical density	0.38 ± 0.02	0.41 ± 0.02	0.01
Diameter of follicles (mm)	2.04 ± 0.64	1.60 ± 0.22	0.001
Circularity of follicles	0.89 ± 0.06	0.91 ± 0.06	0.43
Ferret diameter (mm)	0.75 ± 0.10	0.59 ± 0.08	0.001
Integrated optical density	0.12 ± 0.03	0.08 ± 0.02	0.001

Morphometry of germinative centers of lymph follicles also confirmed higher values of parameters in TH, than in RT (Table 4.).

Table. 4. Quantification of germinative centers (mean ± standard deviation) in tonsillar hypertrophy (TH) and recurrent tonsillitis (RT).

PARAMETERS	TH	RT	$p <$
Areal (mm^2)	0.19 ± 0.08	0.10 ± 0.04	0.001
Optical density	0.35 ± 0.10	0.36 ± 0.07	0.87
Diameter of follicles (mm)	1.60 ± 0.31	1.13 ± 0.17	0.001
Circularity of follicles	0.89 ± 0.05	0.86 ± 0.05	0.96
Ferret diameter (mm)	0.59 ± 0.14	0.42 ± 0.08	0.001
Integrated optical density	0.07 ± 0.02	0.04 ± 0.01	0.001

Discussion

In this study the distribution of TNF-α producing cells was mainly subepithelial, and in germinative centers, while in crypt epithelium and mantle areas they were rare. This is similar to other papers [6, 14]. Contrary to this, some investigators consider verification of intracytoplasmatic cytokines in tonsils very difficult, [10] others found cytokines mainly in mantle areas and extrafollicularly [15]. The differences in distribution of cytokines in palatine tonsils can be attributed to different methods for verification of cytokine producing cells, with unequal specificity and sensitivity [10, 16].

Since the distribution of TNF-α producing cells was similar in TH and RT, quantification was very important for detection of mutual differences. Measurements of N_A and N_V confirmed that TNF-α producing cells were in 55% in subepithelial areas, in 30% in germinative centers, in 13% in interfollicular areas, and in 2% in crypt epithelium in both analyzed groups of chronic tonsillitis. Semiquantitative study of Agren et al, (1995, 1996) [5, 6] found their predomination in germinative centers with bigger number in RT than in TH, as in our study.

Since cytokines are locally produced on the site of infection, the distribution of TNF-α production cells in different morphological compartments of palatine tonsils can contribute to better understanding of immune reactions duing antigen stimulation in chronic tonsillitis.

Immune reaction is initiated in crypt epithelium, so it is infiltrated with B lymphocytes, and less with T lymphocytes, mostly CD4+ cells [17]. Intraepithelial localization of TNF-α producing cells correspond to activated T lymphocytes and macrophages (their production by B cells was not documented). Ageing [18] and chronic tonsillitis [19, 20] cause change in distribution of intraepithelial lymphocytes, what may explain the differences between some authors.

Predomination of TNF-α producing cells in subepithelial areas, found in our study, and in some other studies[6] confirms that subepithelial regions represent the site for contact of antigens and immunocompetent cells [21]. Numerous T lymphocytes, mainly CD4+, are present there, migrating from extrafollicular areas towards crypt epithelium [22]. IgA and IgG producing cells are also localized subepithelially, indicating possible role of TNF-α for producing other cytokines important for differentiation and secretion of Ig-producing cells. It is supposed that TNF-α stimulate clonal selection of activated CD4+ lymphocytes with subsequent influence on cellular, and indirectly on humoral immunity [23, 24]. Since TH usually lacks signs of inflammation, TNF-α in TH is reduced compared to RT [11, 23, 24].

Extrafollicular areas besides T lymphocytes contain interdigitant dendritic cells, B lymphocytes, and plasma cells, representing the site of interaction of Th cells, antigen presenting cells, and B lymphocytes [23]. The presence of TNF-α cells, both in TH and in RT, indicates their role in producing activated Th cells.

Recent studies confirmed that in the beginning of tonsillar inflammation TNF-α are produced by Th1 cells and activated macrophages [25]. Macrophages and dendritic cells are universally present in palatine tonsils, but localization in germinative centers is characteristic for hyperplastic follicles in TH. [24] The role of macrophages in germinative centers of lymph follicles is preominantly in phagocytosis of apoptotic cells, mainly centrocytes that failed clonal selection during differentiation in plasma cells [19, 23]. Thus, the presence of numerous TNF-α producing cells in germinative centers can represent activated macrophages, and Th cells. Ring like distribution of TNF-α cells on the border of germinative center and mantle area corresponds to Th cells and follicular dendritic cells [19].

We found no significant difference in numeric density of TNF-α producing cells in germinative centers in TH and RT group, although morphometry indicated on significantly bigger lymph follicles (areal and circumference) in TH, compared to RT. Similar values of numerical density of TNF-α cells in TH and RT suggest that tonsils in RT retain immunological competence. The presence of abundant TNF-α cells in germinative centers confirms their activity, and immune response to specific antigen. This was also found in other studies, [3] where Th cells and follicular dendritic cells in germinative centers produce many cytokines, TNF-α as well, with stimulation of differentiation of B cells.

Frequent microbial causes of RT are streptococcus pyogenes and hemophylus influenzae. It was documented that membrane M protein from streptococcus pyogenes strongly stimulates TNF-α production [10, 26] Thus, bigger number of TNF-α producing cells in RT can be explained by constant antigen stimulation and inflammation. Contrary to this, TH affects younger population, without morphological signs of inflammation [11].

Recent studies have confirmed that antigen stimulation and mitogen cause increased cytokine formation, primarily TNF-α, interferon-γ, and interleukin 6 [6, 13]. TNF-α production is higher in RT, then in TH, both in our, and in other investigations [5, 25, 26].

Conclusion

Distribution of TNF-α producing cells is similar for TH and RT. They are mainly found in subepithelial areas, interfollicular regions, and germinative centers of lymph follicles, and rarely in crypt epithelium. Numerical density of

TNF-α producing cells is significantly higher in RT, compared to TH. This data confirm domination of cellular Th1 immune response both in TH and RT.

References

[1]   Rink L, Kirchner H. Recent progress in the tumor necrosis factor-alfa field. *Int Archives of Allergy and Immunol* 1996; 111: 199-209.

[2]   Strieter R, Kunkel S, Bone R. Role of tumor necrosis factor-Alfa in disease states and inflammation. *Critical Care Medicine* 1993; 21 (Suppl 10): S447-S463.

[3]   Toellner KM, Toellner DS, Sprenger R, Duchrow M, Trumper LH, Ernst M, Flad HD, Gerdes J. The human germinal centre cells, follicular dendritic cells and germinal centre T cells produce B cell-stimulating cytokines. *Cytokine* 1995; 7: 334-354.

[4]   Tsunoda R, Cormann N, Heinen E, Onozaki K, Coulie P, Akiyama Y, Yoshizaki K, Kinet-Denoel C, Simar LJ, Kojima M. Cytokine produced in lymph follicles. *Immunol Lett* 1989; 22: 129-134.

[5]   Agren K, Andersson U, Nordlander B, Nord CE, Lindae A, Ernberg I, Andersson J. Upregulated local cytokine production in recurrent tonsillitis compared with tonsillar hypertrophy. *Acta Otolaryngol* (Stockh) 1995; 115: 689-696.

[6]   Agren K, Andersson U, Litton M, Funa K, Nordlander B, Andersson J. The production of immunoregulatory cytokines is localised to the extrafollicular area of human tonsils. *Acta Otolaryngol* (Stockh) 1996; 116: 477-485.

[7]   Passali D, Damiani V, Passali GC, Passali FM, Boccayyi A, Bellussi L. Structural and immunological characteristics of chronically inflamed adenotonsillara tissue in chidhood. *Clin Diagn Lab Immunol* 2004; 11: 1154-1157.

[8]   Rostaing L, Tkaczuk J, Durand M, Peres C, Durand D, de Preval C, Ohayon E, Abbal M. Kinetics of intracytoplasmic Th1 and Th2 cytokine production assessed by flow cytometry following in vitro activation of peripheral blood mononuclear cells. *Cytometry* 1999; 35: 318-328.

[9]   Komorowska A, Komorowski J, Banasik M, Lewkowicz P, Tchorsewski H. Cytokines locally produced by lymphocytes removed from the hypertrophic nasopharyngeal and palatine tonsils. *Int J Pediatr Otorhinolaryngol* 2005; 69: 937-941.

[10] Kerakawauchi H, Kurano Y, Mogi G. Immune response against streptococus piogenes in human palatine tonsil. *Laryngoscope* 1997; 107: 634-639.

[11] Surjan L, Brandtzaeg P, Berdal P. Immunoglobulin systems of human tonsilla II. Patients with chronic tonsillitis or tonsillar hyperplasia: quantification of Ig-producing cells, tonsillar morphometry and serum Ig concentrations. *Clin Exp Immunol* 1978; 31: 382-390.

[12] Rhodes A, Miller KD. Internal quality control and external quality assessment of immunocytochemistry. In: *Theory and practice of histological techniques*, bancroft J, Gamble M (eds), fifth edition, Churchill Livingstone, London, UK, 2002, pp 465-498.

[13] Kalisnik M, Vraspir-Porenta O, Kham-Lindtner T, Logonder-Mlinsek M, Pajer Z, Stiblar-Martincic D, Zorc-Pleskovic R, Trobina M: The interdependence of the follicular, parafollicular, and mast cells in the mammalian thyroid gland: a review and a synthesis. *Am J Anat.* 1988;183:148-57.

[14] Andersson J, Andersson U. Characterization of cytokine production in infectious mononucleosis studied at a single-cell level in tonsil and peripheral blood. *Clin Exp Immunol* 1993; 92: 713.

[15] Hoefakker S, van'Erve EH, Deen C, van den Eertwegh AJ, Boersma WJ, Notten WR, Claassen E. Immunohistochemical detection of co-localizing cytokine and antibody producing cells in the extrafollicular area of human palatine tonsils. *Clin Exp Immunol* 1993; 93: 223-228.

[16] Andersson J, Abrams J, Bjork L, Funa K, Litton M, Agren K, Andersson U. Concomitant in vivo production of 19 different cytokines in human tonsils *Immunology* 1994; 83: 16-24.

[17] Brandtzaeg P, Surjan Jr, Berdal P. Immunoglobulin systems of human tonsils I. Control subjects of various ages: quantification of Ig producing cells, tonsillar morphometry and serum concentrations. *Clin Exp Immunol* 1978; 31: 367-381.

[18] Bergler W, Adam S, Gross HJ, Hormann K, Schwartz-Albiez R. Age-dependent altered proportions in subpopulations of tonsillar lymphocytes. *Clin Exp Immunol* 1999; 116: 9-18.

[19] Perry ME. The specialised structure of crypt epithelium in the human palatine tonsil and its functional significance. *J Anat* 1994; 185: 111-127.

[20] Lopez-Gonzales MA, Sanchez B, Mata F, Delgado F. Tonsillar lymphocyte subsets in recurrent acute tonsillitis and tonsillar hypertrophy. *Int J Pediatric Otorhinolaryngol* 1998; 43: 33-39.

[21] Spencer J, Perry ME, Dunn-Walters DK. Human marginal – zone B cells. *Immunol Today* 1998; 19: 421-426.

[22] Favre A, Poletti M, Marzoli A, Pesce G, Giampalmo A, Rossi F. The human palatine tonsil studied from surgical specimens at all ages and various pathological conditions. *Z Mikrosk Anat Forsch* 1986; 100: 7-33.

[23] Brandtzaeg P. Immunology of tonsils and adenoids: everything the ENT surgeon needs to know. *Int J Pediatric Otorhinolaryngol* 2003; 6751: 569-576.

[24] Avramović V, Vlahović P, Savić V, Stanković M. Localisation of ecto 5' nucleotidase and divalent cation activated ecto ATP-ase in chronic tonsillitis. *ORL* 1998; 60: 174-177.

[25] Wakashima j, Harabuchi Y, Shirasaki H. *A study of cytokine in palatine tonsil-cytokine mRNA expression determined by RT-PCR.* Nippon Jibiinkoka Gakkai Kaiho 1999; 102: 254-264.

[26] Agren K, Brauner A, Andersson J. Haemophilus influencae and streptococcus puogenes group A challenge induce a Th1 type of cytokine response in cells obtained from tonsillar hypertrophy and recurrent tonsillitis. *ORL* 1998; 60: 35-41.

In: Tonsillar Disorders
Editor: Anne C. Hallberg

ISBN: 978-1-61209-275-1
©2011 Nova Science Publishers, Inc.

Short Communication

Peritonsillar Abscess*

Olaf Zagólski

Diagnostic and Therapeutic Medical Centre 'Medicina',
ENT Department, Kraków, Poland

Abstract

Peritonsillar abscess (quinsy) is a complication of acute bacterial tonsillitis. Its treatment remains controversial. Needle drainage of the abscess may provide an alternative to incision or tonsillectomy. An important element of controversy is the choice of antibiotics after surgical drainage of the abscess. Results of many studies support the resistance of grown bacteria to many antibiotics and the potential importance of anaerobic bacteria in development of peritonsillar abscesses. Although bacteria grown from the pus vary among the continents, clinical implications resulting from the microbiological studies are similar. Patients with peritonsillar abscesses should be treated with antibiotics effective against both aerobic and anaerobic bacteria.

In the routine management of peritonsillar abscess, bacteriologic studies are unnecessary on initial presentation. It is, however, necessary to consider infection with anaerobes. Therefore, penicillin and

---

* A version of this chapter was also published in *Handbook of Pharyngeal Diseases: Etiology, Diagnosis and Treatment,* edited by Aaron P. Nazario and Julien K. Vermeulen, published by Nova Science Publishers, Inc. It was submitted for appropriate modifications in an effort to encourage wider dissemination of research.

metronidazole are recommended as the antibiotic regimen of choice in the treatment of peritonsillar abscesses. If this treatment is ineffective, broad-spectrum antibiotics (clinadmycin) should be administered.

Introduction

Peritonsillar abscess (quinsy) is a reservoir of pus collected in the peritonsillar space, limited by the superior pharyngeal sphincter and the capsule of the tonsil [1], developing as a complication of bacterial tonsillitis [2, 3, 4]. Most rise secondary to an oropharyngeal or dental infection. Additional factors, such as smoking and periodontal disease, may also contribute to the formation of a peritonsillar abscess [3, 5]. The disease is in the majority of cases unilateral [6]. Diagnosis is clinical—in doubtful cases confirmed with biopsy or computed tomography [3, 7]. When no pus is identified on incision and drainage, the diagnosis of peritonsillar cellulitis is established [8]. The estimated annual incidence of peritonsillar abscesses is 30 cases per 100,000 inhabitants [9, 10]. Currently, less than 20 % of all peritonsillar infections occur in the pediatric population. [7, 11, 12]. About 10% of peritonsillar abscesses recur [9]. The true incidence of bilateral peritonsillar abscesses is unknown, but the incidence of unsuspected contralateral peritonsillar abscess identified at tonsillectomy has been reported to be between 1.9% and 24% [6]. The diagnosis of bilateral peritonsillar abscesses should be considered when the clinical presentation suggests the diagnosis of peritonsillar abscess, but the physical examination reveals bilateral swollen tonsils with a midline uvula [6]. The fact that peritonsillar abscesses develop only in some patients, still has to be explained. Many pus samples contain inflammatory cells in abundance but they are mostly deformed and only occasionally can intracellular bacteria be recognized. Insufficient immunoglobulin-coating of bacteria might be an important aetiopathogenic factor in the development of a peritonsillar abscess [13].

Treatment of Peritonsillar Abscess

The treatment of peritonsillar abscess remains controversial [14]. Adequate drainage with accompanying antimicrobial therapy and hydration are the cornerstones of management. Catheter or needle drainage of these abscesses may provide an alternative to open procedures and is the drainage method of choice for peritonsillar abscesses. There is also a limited but useful place for immediate tonsillectomy in the treatment of this disease [3, 9, 15]. The presumption that the abscess can be drained not only by otorhinolaryngologists, but also by general or emergency care specialists should be verified by the close proximity of the internal carotid artery—a distance of about 1 cm from the tonsillar capsule [9]. Peritonsillar abscess can be successfully treated by three-point puncture and aspiration. The results (recurrence in 19%) are comparable with published data on drainage of the peritonsillar space through the incision procedure. If the bacterial culture shows mixed aerobic and anaerobic flora, but not S. pyogenes, and if the patient has a history of recurrent tonsillitis, incision or proceeding directly to tonsillectomy may be the best therapeutic choice [1]. An important element of controversy is the choice of antibiotics after surgical drainage of the abscess [14]. Intramuscular or intravenous route is used [16]. Antibiotics prevent spread of the infection, which leads to a descending process with consecutive mediastinitis and/or sepsis as a life-threatening condition [4]. Antibiotic therapy started for tonsillitis does not prevent the occurrence of peritonsillar abscess in 45% of patients and has no influence on the clinical course of the disease [2]. However, in selected cases, medical therapy alone, especially in children, can resolve parapharyngeal and hypopharyngeal abscesses [3]. Ancillary use of steroids reduces morbidity in patients with a peritonsillar abscess [3, 7]. Admission to the hospital is not always necessary if a correct outpatient control is possible [10]. Proper hydration, oral and in some cases intravenous, is necessary as some patients may develop dysphagia [17].

Obtaining Pus for Microbiological Examination

Proper management of the material from peritonsillar abscesses is very important to establish the pathogen and it should be obtained by aspiration in order to prevent contamination with nasopharyngeal and throat bacteria [18, 19]. At least 3 ml of pus are required [20]. The material for aerobic culture should be transferred to transport basis. Pus to be cultured for anaerobic bacteria must be sent to the laboratory immediately after aspiration in a hermetically closed syringe [20, 21].

Bacteriology of Peritonsillar Abscesses

Streptococcus pyogenes (Group A beta-streptococcus) is commonly considered an important pathogen in this infection [22]. However, recent studies have demonstrated the recovery of many other streptococci mainly consisting of alpha-streptococci [22]. As antibiotics are being used widely, normal flora such as the Streptococcus milleri group has become an important pathogen in peritonsillar abscesses due to an imbalance between organisms and host defense [22]. The Streptococcus milleri group, consisting of 3 species of Streptococcus constellatus, Streptococcus intermedius, and Streptococcus anginosus, forms part of the normal flora most commonly found in the mouth, throat, gastrointestinal tract, and genital tract. These species have become known as an important pathogen in abscess disease but little attention has been paid to their role in peritonsillar abscesses [22]. Many authors stress the importance of anaerobic bacteria in development of peritonsillar abscesses, both in mixed flora and as exclusive agents [13, 18, 19, 22, 23, 24]. Some anaerobic bacteria possess interfering capability with Group A beta-hemolytic streptococci and other pathogens [23]. Peritonsillar abscesses containing beta-haemolytic streptococci Group A, which appear as a single species, contain fewer bacteria per ml than effusions harboring a mixed flora [25]. The possible role of anaerobes in the acute inflammatory process in the tonsils is supported by several observations: anaerobes have been isolated from the cores of tonsils in patients with recurrent Group A beta-hemolytic streptococcal and non-Group A beta-hemolytic streptococcal tonsillitis; the recovery of anaerobes as predominant pathogens in abscesses of tonsils, in many cases without any aerobic bacteria; their recovery as pathogens in well-established anaerobic infections of the tonsils (Vincent's angina), and of their neck complications [23]. Haeggstrom et al. [19] established that all bacteria isolated from peritonsillar abscesses were susceptible to penicillin V, ampicillin and erythromycin when tested in vitro, as some anaerobic bacteria are sensitive to penicillin. However, sensitivity in vitro does not always reflect sensitivity in vivo [19]. Cherukuri et al. [26] observed that the majority of grew organisms were penicillin-resistant. Only a limited number of microbiological studies assessing the bacterial flora of peritonsillar abscesses has been performed and their results seem contradictory [13, 18, 19, 22, 23]. The differences might mainly result from diversity of the bacterial flora in different regions of the world.

Differences of Bacterial Flora of Peritonsillar Abscesses in Different Regions of the World

The results of bacteriological studies presented by several authors differ considerably.

In the USA, Brook et al. [18] analyzed 34 peritonsillar abscesses. A total 107 bacterial isolates (58 anaerobic, and 49 aerobic and facultative) were recovered, accounting for 3.1 isolates per specimen (1.7 anaerobic, and 1.4 aerobic and facultatives). Anaerobic bacteria only were present in 6 (18%) patients, aerobic and facultatives in 2 (6%), and mixed aerobic and anaerobic flora in 26 (76%). Single bacterial isolates were recovered in 4 infections, 2 of which were Streptococcus pyogenes and 2 were anaerobic bacteria. The predominant bacterial isolates were Staphylococcus aureus (6 isolates), Bacteroides sp. (21 isolates, including 15 Bacteroides melaninogenicus group), and Peptostreptococcus sp. (16) and Streptococcus pyogenes (10). Beta-Lactamase-producing organisms were recovered from 13 (52%) of 25 specimens tested.

In Scandinavia, Haeggstrom et al. [6] tested abscess material from 10 patients with peritonsillar abscesses. A total of 26 bacterial species were isolated from the abscess material; 19 of these were obligate anaerobes. In 4 patients a pure growth of anaerobes was found. In 3 patients a mixed aerobe/anaerobe flora was obtained. In 3 patients a pure growth of aerobes was found. Beta-hemolytic streptococci groups A and C respectively were isolated from 2 patients, but in pure culture from one patient only.

In Japan, Fujiyoshi et al. [22] performed bacteriological examination in 31 cases of peritonsillar abscess. The Streptococcus milleri group was most frequently isolated (25.8%), followed by Eikenella corrodens (9.7%), Staphylococcus aureus (6.5%), and Streptococcus pyogenes (3.2%).

In Great Britain, Prior et al. [24] examined pus from 53 peritonsillar. A positive culture grew in 85% of quinsies and of these 16% produced aerobes and 84% anaerobes. Penicillin-resistant organisms were grown from 32% of patients and all but one of these organisms (Haemophilus influenzae) was sensitive to metronidazole. The effectiveness of penicillin and metronidazole as the antibiotic regimen of choice in the treatment of peritonsillar abscesses was confirmed in 98% of patients.

Sakae et al. [20] examined 39 patients with peritonsillar abscesses. 34 (87%) samples showed positive cultures. Aerobic or facultative aerobic bacteria were isolated from 9 aspirates, mixed aerobic and anaerobic bacteria from 24, and anaerobic bacteria from only 1 aspirate. A total of 69 bacterial isolates (34 aerobic and 35 anaerobic) were recovered. The most common aerobic isolate was Streptococcus sp., with Streptococcus pyogenes being identified in 23% of aspirates. The predominant anaerobic isolates were Prevotella sp. and Peptostreptococcus sp.

Conclusion

Results of the presented studies from various countries confirm that bacterial flora of the peritonsillar abscesses varies between the continents, although clinical conclusions deriving from them are convergent. A comparison of two groups of patients: 58 patients treated with broad-spectrum intravenous antibiotics and 45 patients treated with intravenous penicillin alone, after drainage of the abscess, disclosed that clinical outcomes with respect to hours hospitalized and mean hours febrile were not statistically significantly different between the groups [14]. This indicates that broad-spectrum antibiotics fail to show greater efficacy than penicillin in the treatment of these patients. These results suggest that intravenous penicillin remains an excellent choice for therapy in cases of peritonsillar abscess requiring parenteral antibiotics after drainage [14]. In the cited studies, the obtained aerobic bacteria were usually sensitive to oral penicillin (phenoxymethylpenicillin) [7, 24]. However, in some patients, pathogens resistant to penicillin were also found [24, 26]. Therefore, due to a high probability of infection with anaerobic bacteria, it seems reasonable to administer metronidazole from the beginning of the therapy in all patients with peritonsillar abscess who do not report contraindications to such a regime [24]. The author's clinical experience confirms that some of the anaerobic bacteria within pus obtained from peritonsillar abscesses are resistant to metronidazole and sensitive to penicillin and some aerobic bacteria are resistant to penicillin and sensitive to metronidazole. It must be remembered that a high prevalence of penicillin allergy has been reported in patients with peritonsillar abscess [8]. The majority of the infections are resolved by administration of penicillin with metronidazole. In resistant cases a broad-spectrum anaerobic antibiotic (e.g., clindamycin) should be subsequently added [7, 16]. Bacteriologic studies are not necessary in the routine management of peritonsillitis [10, 17]. They should be reserved for patients with a high likelihood of infection by resistant organisms, i.e., diabetics, immunocompromised patients, patients with recurrent peritonsillar abscess, and in cases of further development of the purulent infiltration [26]. It is important to remember that culture for anaerobic bacteria takes up to 10 days.

References

[1] Savolainen, S; Jousimies-Somer, HR; Makitie, AA; Ylikoski, JS. Peritonsillar abscess. Clinical and microbiologic aspects and treatment regimens. *Arch Otolaryngol Head Neck Surg,* 1993, 119, 521-524.

[2] Briner, HR. Does antibiotic therapy hinder the course of peritonsillar abscesses? *Schweiz Med Wochenschr,* 2000, 125, 14S-16S.

[3] Herzon, FS; Martin, AD. Medical and surgical treatment of peritonsillar, retropharyngeal, and parapharyngeal abscesses. *Curr Infect Dis Rep,* 2006, 8, 196-202.

[4] Kinzer, S; Maier, W; Ridder, GJ. Abscess: a Lifethreatening Disease - Diagnostic and Therapeutic Aspects. *Laryngorhinootologie,* 2007, 86, 371-375.

[5] Lehnerdt, G; Senska, K; Fischer, M. Smoking promotes the formation of peritonsillar abscesses. *Laryngorhinootologie,* 2005, 84, 676-679.

[6] Fasano, CJ; Chudnofsky, C; Vanderbeek, P. Bilateral peritonsillar abscesses: not your usual sore throat. *J Emerg Med,* 2005, 29, 45-47.

[7] Garcia, Callejo FJ; Nunez Gomez, F; Sala Franco, J; Marco Algarra, J. Management of peritonsillar infections. *An Pediatr (Barc),* 2006, 65, 37-43.

[8] Chandra, RK; Lee, CE; Pelzer, H. Prevalence of penicillin allergy in adults with peritonsillar abscess. *Ear Nose Throat J,* 2005, 84, 234-236.

[9] Herzon, FS. Harris P. Mosher Award thesis. Peritonsillar abscess: incidence, current management practices, and a proposal for treatment guidelines. *Laryngoscope* 1995, 3 Suppl, 1-17.

[10] Palomar Asenjo, V; Borras Perera, M; Ruiz Giner, A; Palomar Garcia, V. Peritonsillar infection. Out-patient management. *An Otorrinolaringol Ibero Am,* 2006, 33, 399-407.

[11] Herzon, FS; Nicklaus, P. Pediatric peritonsillar abscess: management guidelines. *Curr Probl Pediatr,* 1996, 26, 270-278.

[12] Hromadkova, P. Peritonsillar abscess in children. *Bratisl Lek Listy,* 2006, 107, 272-275.

[13] Lilja, M; Raisanen, S; Stenfors, LE. Immunoglobulin- and complement-coated bacteria in pus from peritonsillar abscesses. *J Laryngol Otol,* 1998, 112, 634-638.

[14] Kieff, DA; Bhattacharyya, N; Siegel, NS; Salman, SD. Selection of antibiotics after incision and drainage of peritonsillar abscesses. *Otolaryngol Head Neck Surg,* 1999, 120, 57-61.

[15] Khayr, W; Taepke, J. Management of peritonsillar abscess: needle aspiration versus incision and drainage versus tonsillectomy. *Am J Ther,* 2005, 12, 344-350.

[16] Ozbek, C; Aygenc, E; Unsal, E; Ozdem, C. Peritonsillar abscess: a comparison of outpatient i.m. clindamycin and inpatient i.v. ampicillin/sulbactam following needle aspiration. *Ear Nose Throat J,* 2005, 84, 366-368.

[17] Lamkin, RH; Portt, J. An outpatient medical treatment protocol for peritonsillar abscess. *Ear Nose Throat J,* 2006, 85, 660-667.

[18] Brook, I; Frazier, EH; Thompson, DH. Aerobic and anaerobic microbiology of peritonsillar abscess. *Laryngoscope,* 1991, 101, 289-292.

[19] Haeggstrom, A; Engquist, S; Hallander H. Bacteriology in peritonsillitis. *Acta Otolaryngol,* 1987, 103, 151-155.

[20] Sakae, FA; Imamura, R; Sennes, LU; Araujo Filho, BC; Tsuji, DH . Microbiology of peritonsillar abscesses. *Rev Bras Otorrinolaringol,* 2006, 72, 247-251.

[21] Badran, K. How to avoid spillage of pus when draining peritonsillar abscess. *Clin Otolaryngol,* 2005, 30, 567-568.

[22] Fujiyoshi, T; Inaba, T; Udaka, T; Tanabe, T; Yoshida, M; Makishima, K. Clinical significance of the Streptococcus milleri group in peritonsillar abscesses. *Nippon Jibiinkoka Gakkai Kaiho,* 2001, 104, 866-871.

[23] Brook, I. The role of anaerobic bacteria in tonsillitis. *Int J Pediatr Otorhinolaryngol,* 2005, 69, 9-19.

[24] Prior, A; Montgomery, P; Mitchelmore, I; Tabaqchali, S. The microbiology and antibiotic treatment of peritonsillar abscesses. *Clin Otolaryngol Allied Sci,* 1995, 20, 219-223.

[25] Lilja, M; Raianen, S; Jokinen, K; Stenfors, LE. Direct microscopy of effusions obtained from peritonsillar abscesses as a complement to bacterial culturing. *J Laryngol Otol,* 1997, 111, 392-395.

[26] Cherukuri, S; Benninger, MS. Use of bacteriologic studies in the outpatient management of peritonsillar abscess. *Laryngoscope,* 2002, 112, 18-20.

Index

immunoglobulin, viii, 8, 17, 21, 25, 33, 36, 49, 79, 92
immunoglobulins, 15, 45, 46, 47, 48, 49
immunohistochemistry, 37
immunomodulatory, 55
immunostimulant, 48, 49, 50
immunotherapy, vii, ix, 40, 41, 45, 47, 48, 49
in vitro, 8, 88, 94
in vivo, 2, 89, 94
incidence, 5, 9, 15, 18, 19, 43, 46, 47, 68, 73, 74, 92, 97
individuals, x, 17, 46, 67
infancy, viii, 2
infants, 4, 6, 11, 60
infection, viii, ix, x, xi, 2, 6, 7, 10, 13, 39, 40, 41, 42, 43, 44, 45, 46, 47, 50, 51, 53, 56, 57, 58, 60, 61, 62, 67, 71, 74, 76, 79, 86, 91, 92, 93, 94, 96, 97
infectious mononucleosis, 89
inflammation, viii, 2, 4, 6, 7, 8, 13, 50, 56, 57, 61, 64, 86, 87, 88
inflammatory cells, 92
influenza, 57
influenza virus, 57
insertion, 5, 10, 18
institutions, 68
integrated optical density (IOD), x, 78, 80
intensive care unit, 11, 19
interdependence, 89
interference, 52
interferon, 79, 87
interferon-γ, 79, 87
intervention, 10, 70
intima, 37
intramuscular injection, 43
intravenous antibiotics, 96
involution, 2
irrigation, 18
Italy, 1, 39

J

Japan, 95
joints, 56

K

kill, 48
killer cells, 48

L

laboratory tests, 79
lead, ix, 7, 24, 39, 43, 44, 64
lesions, 41, 42
leukemia, 60
light, 23, 27, 28, 32, 34, 61
local anesthesia, 69, 73
local anesthetic, 62
localization, viii, 3, 22, 28, 32, 33, 34, 80, 86, 87
low risk, 11, 69
lymph, ix, x, 39, 40, 54, 78, 80, 82, 83, 85, 87, 88
lymph gland, ix, 39, 40
lymphocytes, viii, 2, 3, 7, 22, 25, 26, 31, 32, 33, 34, 36, 37, 48, 49, 55, 86, 88, 89
lymphoid, vii, viii, ix, 2, 3, 4, 7, 13, 15, 17, 21, 22, 23, 24, 25, 26, 27, 28, 30, 31, 32, 33, 34, 35, 36, 37, 39, 40, 47, 48, 49, 50, 54
lymphoid follicle, vii, viii, 21, 22, 23, 24, 25, 26, 27, 28, 30, 32, 33, 34, 35, 54
lymphoid follicle function, vii
lymphoid organs, 34
lymphoid tissue, ix, 2, 3, 7, 13, 15, 26, 28, 30, 39, 40, 47, 48, 49, 50, 54
lymphoma, 37
lysozyme, 3

M

machinery, 52
macrophages, 7, 27, 46, 47, 48, 78, 86, 87
magnesium, 24
majority, 92, 94, 96
management, vii, ix, xi, 1, 5, 10, 40, 41, 51, 68, 72, 75, 91, 92, 93, 96, 97, 99
mantle, viii, 22, 25, 26, 27, 28, 29, 31, 33, 34, 35, 54, 81, 82, 83, 85, 87
mast cells, vii, 2, 7, 8, 13, 17, 18, 89

U

V

W

X

Y